2

140 Must Know Meds
Demolish Nursing Pharmacology

NRSNG.com|NursingStudentBooks.com

Jon Haws RN CCRN
Tarang Patel RN CCRN RPh
Kati Kleber RN CCRN

Based on the "MedMaster" Podcast by NRSNG.com

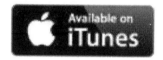

4

As a Gift:

http://www.nrsng.com/50meds

Wonder which are the most commonly prescribed medications?

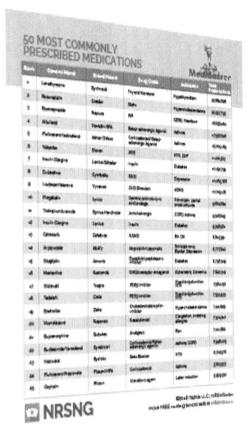

Download our free PDF cheat sheet covering the 50 Most Commonly Prescribed Medications

Just visit NRSNG.com/50meds

How to use this book:

This book is divided into two sections; individual medications and medication classes. Under the individual medications you will find the most important information you need to know about the given medication to pass tests and provide safe patient care. This **is not to be considered** a complete list of all considerations for the medications but simply a guide to help you learn the MOST important tested information. The medication class section covers some of the most often tested medication classes and should be used to learn the general basics of some of the most common classes.

Contents

Introduction

This book is based on the Med of the Day Podcast and is part of the MedMaster Course.

I remember my first day as a sophomore nursing student in Nursing Pharmacology. To say I was lost is an understatement. It was like someone had dropped me off in a completely foreign land with an incomprehensible language. When I entered nursing school the only real health care experience I had was working as a transporter in a large hospital. Pharmacology was new to me and I was terrified that I would never be able to grasp the lingo.

The good news was my study partner had actually attended pharmacy school in India before coming to the United States to study nursing. The bad news was the **Pharmacology makes up about 15% of the questions on the NCLEX®** and I only had a semester to learn it!

The next few months were spent intently studying and taking practice exams. During the course of taking countless practice exams I would jot down every medication that was tested. I also would jot down the fact about the specific medication or class that was being tested.

This book is a compilation of the 140 must know meds for the NCLEX® and Nursing Pharmacology. These medications were the most tested. While the nursing considerations listed are not complete (and are not intended to be) they contain the most frequently tested material that you need to know for a given medication.

If you can learn the key facts about these medications you will ace your course and the NCLEX. The fact that you have downloaded this book proves that you are serious about your nursing career!

Oh yeah! I did end up passing Nursing Pharmacology with an "A" and continue to study pharmacology . . . but now I really enjoy it.

Happy Nursing!

-Jon Haws RN CCRN

NRSNG.com | NursingStudentBooks.com | MedMasterCourse.com

17

About the Authors

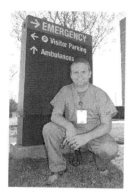

Jon Haws RN BSN CCRN - Having worked as an ICU nurse, preceptor, Code Team Nurse, ICU Charge Nurse, and mentor to thousands of nursing students I strive give you the support, encouragement, education, and tools you need to succeed in nursing school, pass the NCLEX, and excel as a nurse. I have a relentless passion for simplifying the process of nursing education. . . it has become unnecessarily over-complicated, with too much fluff and politics. It's time to ditch the old way.

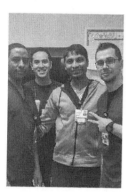

Tarang Patel RN BSN CCRN RPh - Tarang is a Pharmacist, Critical Care RN, and Nurse Anesthetist student allowing him to bring a unique perspective to nursing education. Having working in the several ICUs as a staff nurse, agency, travel nurse, and precepting scores of students and new nurses, Tarang knows what it takes to succeed on the floor.

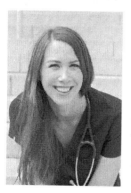

Kati Kleber RN BSN CCRN - I am a bedside nurse and have been since I graduated. I've work on the floor, step-down and in critical care. I have my bachelor's degree that I received in 2010 and am nationally certified. I still work with patients and other nurses on the front lines. Because of this, I am aware of the ever-evolving challenges that face the bedside nurse. I know what it takes for students to be successful at the bedside because I am still there.

50 Most Commonly Prescribed Med Free Cheatsheet: **NRSNG.com/50meds**
Nursing School Shouldn't be so DAMN Hard!
©2016 TazKai LLC | NRSNG.com

Alteplase

Generic Name

alteplase

Trade Name

t-PA

Indication

MI, acute ischemic stroke, occluded central lines

Action

converts plasminogen to plasmin which degrades the fibrin found in clots

Therapeutic Class

thrombolytics

Pharmacologic Class

plasminogen activators

Nursing Considerations

- contraindicated in active bleeding
- **monitor closely for signs of bleeding (petechiae)**
  - q 15 min X1hr
  - q 15-30 min X 8 hr
- use caution with patient who have had recent surgery
- may cause intracranial hemorrhage
- monitor for anaphylaxis
- use caution with uncontrolled hypertension
- **assess neuro status during therapy**

Atorvastatin

Generic Name

atorvastatin

Trade Name

Lipitor

Indication

management of high cholesterol (hypercholesterolemia), primary prevention of cardiovascular disease

Action

lowers total cholesterol as well as LDL while slightly increasing HDL. Inhibits HMG-CoA reductase which plays a role in the liver in cholesterol formation

Therapeutic Class

lipid-lowering agent

Pharmacologic Class

HMG-CoA reductase inhibitor

Similar Medications

simvistatin (Zocor), rosuvastatin (Crestor)

Nursing Considerations

- contraindicated in active liver disease
- may cause rhabdomyolysis
- monitor renal function
- monitor serum cholesterol before, about 4 weeks after starting, and frequently during drug therapy
- monitor liver function tests

- instruct patient to report muscle weakness (sign of rhabdomyolysis)

Acetaminophen

Generic Name

acetaminophen

Trade Name

Tylenol

Indication

pain, fever

Action

inhibit the synthesis of prostaglandins which play a role in transmission of pain signals and fever response

Therapeutic Class

antipyretic, non-opioid analgesic

Nursing Considerations

- **do not exceed 4g of acetaminophen per day to limit risk for liver, renal, and cardiac damage**
- overdose will lead to hepatotoxicity
- Acetadote is the antidote for overdose
- may increase risk for bleed with warfarin therapy
- may alter blood glucose measurements

Acyclovir

Generic Name

acyclovir

Trade Name

Zovirax

Indication

genital herpes, herpes zoster, chicken pox

Action

interferes with viral DNA synthesis

Therapeutic Class

antiviral

Pharmacologic Class

purine analogues

Nursing Considerations

- may cause seizures, renal failure, Stevens-Johnson syndrome, thrombotic thrombocytopenic purpura syndrome, diarrhea, dizziness, nausea
- monitor renal panel during administration
- assess lesions
- instruct patient to use proper protection during sexual intercourse

Albuterol

Generic Name

albuterol

Trade Name

Proventil

Indication

bronchodilator used to prevent airway obstruction in asthma and COPD

Action

binds to Beta2 adrenergic receptors in the airway leading to relaxation of the smooth muscles in the airways

Therapeutic Class

bronchodilator

Pharmacologic Class

adrenergic

Nursing Considerations

- may decrease the effectiveness of Beta Blockers
- use caution with
  - heart disease
  - diabetes
  - glaucoma
  - seizure disorder
- overuse of inhalers can lead to bronchospasm
- monitor for chest pain and palpitations
- can decrease digoxin levels

Alendronate

Generic Name

alendronate

Trade Name

Fosamax

Indication

osteoporosis (aging, menopause, corticosteroid induced)

Action

inhibits osteoclast activity leading to inhibition of resorption of bone

Therapeutic Class

bone resorption inhibitor

Pharmacologic Class

bisphosphnates

Nursing Considerations

- **take first thing in the morning with full glass of water 30 min prior to eating**
- assess serum calcium and vitamin D
- may lead to muscle pain

Alprazolam

Generic Name

Alprazolam

Trade Name

Xanax

Indication

anxiety, panic disorder, manage symptoms of PMS, insomnia, mania, psychosis

Action

works in CNS to produce anxiolytic effect causing CNS depression.

Therapeutic Class

antianxiety agent

Pharmacologic Class

benzodiazepine

Nursing Considerations

- **use caution with existing CNS depression, sleep apnea, renal dysfunction, hepatic dysfunction.**
- may cause CNS depression, drowsiness, lethargy
- may lead to physical dependence, may experience tolerance effect
- assess anxiety and mental status
- Romazicon (lumazenil) is the antidote for overdose
- Grapefruit juice may increase blood levels

Amiodarone

Generic Name

Amiodarone

Trade Name

Cordarone

Indication

a-fib, ventricular arrhythmias, SVT, ACLS protocol for v-fib and v-tach

Action

prolongs phase 3 of the action potential, makes the heart more tolerant to arrythmias, inhibits adrenergic stimulation, slows rate, decreases peripheral vascular resistance causing vasodilation

Therapeutic Class

antiarrhythmic class III, potassium channel blocker

Pharmacologic Class

Nursing Considerations

- may lead to ARDS, pulmonary toxicity, CHF, bradycardia, hypotension
- **increases risk for QT prolongation**
- increases digoxin levels
- increases activity of warfarin
- monitor EKG continuously while on therapy
- assess for signs and symptoms of ARDS
- monitor liver function test
- check dosage with another RN
- teach pt to monitor pulse daily and report abnormalities
- **avoid drinking grapefruit juice**

Amitryptiline

Generic Name

Amitryptiline

Trade Name

Elavil

Indication

depression, anxiety, insomnia, parkinsons

Action

increases effect of serotonin and norepinephrine in the CNS, exhibits anticholinergic effects

Therapeutic Class

antidepressant

Pharmacologic Class

tricyclic antidepressant

Nursing Considerations

- contraindicated in MI, heart failure, **QT prolongation**, glaucoma
- may increase risk for suicidal ideation
- may cause arrhythmias, hypotension, EKG changes
- may cause alterations in blood glucose levels
- may lead to general sedation and lethargy
- **do not use within 2 weeks of MAOIs**
- Instruct pt to take medication exactly as instructed
- monitor for orthostatic hypotension
- may lead to photosensitivity, instruct patient to use sunscreen
- may turn urine blue/green color.

Amlodipine

Generic Name

Amlodipine

Trade Name

Norvasc

Indication

hypertension, angina

Action

blocks transport of calcium into muscle cells inhibiting excitation and contraction

Therapeutic Class

antihypertensive

Pharmacologic Class

Ca channel blocker

Nursing Considerations

- **may cause gingival hyperplasia**
- grapefruit juice may increase drug level
- monitor blood pressure and pulse prior to and during therapy
- monitor intake and output
- assess for signs of CHF
- **assess characteristics of angina**
- instruct patient of interventions for hypertension and how to take blood pressure

Amoxicillin

Generic Name

amoxicillin

Trade Name

Moxatag

Indication

skin infections, respiratory infections, sinusitis, endocarditis prophylaxis, lyme disease

Action

Inhibits synthesis of bacterial cell wall leading to cell death.

Therapeutic Class

anti-infectives, antiulcer agent

Pharmacologic Class

aminopenicillins

Nursing Considerations

- contraindicated with penicillin allergy
- may cause seizures
- assess for rash, anaphylaxis
- excreted by kidneys - monitor renal labs
- **monitor patient for diarrhea - bloody stool should be reported immediately**

Ampicillin

Generic Name

ampicillin

Trade Name

Principen

Indication

skin infections, soft tissue infections, otitis media, sinusitis, respiratory infections, GU infections, meningitis, septicemia

Action

bactericidal, broader spectrum than penicillin, binds to cell wall leading to bacterial cell death

Therapeutic Class

anti-infective

Pharmacologic Class

aminopenicillin

Nursing Considerations

- **contraindicated in penicillin allergy, use caution in renal insufficiency**
- may lead to seizures, diarrhea, anaphylaxes, super infection
- assess for infection
- monitor liver function tests
- instruct patient on signs of super infection: fury over growth on tongue, vaginal itching, loose and foul smelling stool
- pt should not use with oral contraceptive use.

Aspirin

Generic Name

aspirin

Trade Name

Bayer Aspirin

Indication

rheumatoid arthritis, osteoarthritis, ischemic stroke and MI prophylaxis

Action

inhibits the production of prostaglandins which leads to a reduction of fever and inflammation, decreases platelet aggregation leading to a decrease in ischemic diseases

Therapeutic Class

antipyretics, non-opioid analgesics

Pharmacologic Class

salicylates

Nursing Considerations

- use caution in bleeding disorders, chronic alcohol use
- may lead to Stevens-Johnson syndrome, laryngeal edema, and anaphylaxis
- increases risk for bleeding with warfarin, heparin, and clopidogrel
- increased risk for GI bleeding with NSAID use
- monitor liver function tests
- concurrent use with alcohol may increase risk for GI bleeding
- aspirin with viral infections can cause Reye's syndrome

Atenolol

Generic Name

atenolol

Trade Name

Tenormin

Indication

hypertension, angina, prevention of MI

Action

blocks the stimulation of beta$_1$ receptors in the SNS with minimal effect on beta$_2$ receptors

Therapeutic Class

antianginal, antihypertensive

Pharmacologic Class

beta blocker

Nursing Considerations

- Contraindicated in CHF, pulmonary edema, cardiogenic shock, bradycardia, heart block
- monitor hemodynamic parameters (HR, BP)
- **May cause bradycardia, CHF, pulmonary edema**
- masks symptoms associated with diabetes mellitus
- advise to change positions slowly to prevent orthostatic hypotension
- instruct patient on how to take blood pressure

Atropine

Generic Name

atropine

Trade Name

Atro-pen

Indication

decreases oral and respiratory secretions, treats sinus bradycardia and heart block, treatment of bronchospasm

Action

Atropine is an anticholinergic which means that it inhibits the effects of the parasympathetic nervous system, specifically acetylcholine. This inhibition causes increase in HR, bronchodilation, decreased GI and respiratory secretions.

Therapeutic Class

antiarrhythmic

Pharmacologic Class

anticholinergic, antimuscarinic

Nursing Considerations

- avoid in acute hemorrhage, tachycardia, and angle closure glaucoma
- monitor patient for tachycardia and palpitations
- may cause urinary retention in elderly patients
- patients may experience constipation due to slowed GI motility

Azithromycin

Generic Name

azithromycin

Trade Name

Zithromax

Indication

URI, chronic bronchitis, lower respiratory infections, otitis media, skin infections, various STIs, prevention of bacterial endocarditis, treatment of cystic fibrosis

Action

inhibits bacterial protein synthesis

Therapeutic Class

agents for atypical mycobacterium, anti-infectives

Pharmacologic Class

Macrolide

Nursing Considerations

- may lead to pseudomembranous colitis, pain, diarrhea, nausea, Stevens-Johnson syndrome, angioedema
- may increase risks for warfarin toxicity
- monitor patient for signs of anaphylaxis
- instruct patient to notify physician for diarrhea, or blood or pus in stool
- instruct patient to take medication exactly as prescribed

Benzotropine

Generic Name

benzotropine

Trade Name

Cogentin

Indication

treatment for Parkinson's disease

Action

exhibits anticholinergic properties (blocks acetylcholine) in the CNS to reduce rigidity and tremors

Therapeutic Class

Antiparkinson agent

Pharmacologic Class

Anticholinergic

Nursing Considerations

- may lead to arrhythmias, hypotension, palpitations, and tachycardia
- anticholinergic effects like constipation, dry mouth
- assess for extrapyramidal symptoms
- instruct patient to take as directed
- instruct patient to maintain good oral hygiene

Bisacodyl

Generic Name

bisacodyl

Trade Name

Dulcolax

Indication

treatment of constipation, bowel regimen

Action

stimulates enteric nerves to cause peristalsis which leads to fluid accumulation in the colon

Therapeutic Class

laxatives

Pharmacologic Class

stimulant laxatives

Nursing Considerations

- may lead to hypokalemia
- may cause abdominal pain and cramps
- use caution with milk
- assess for abdominal distention and bowel function
- **instruct patient to drink 1500-2000 mL/day during therapy**
- monitor fluid and electrolyte levels
- instruct patient to take as ordered

Bismuth Subsalicylate

Generic Name

bismuth subsalicylate

Trade Name

Kaopectate, Pepto-Bismol

Indication

diarrhea, heartburn, indigestion, H. pylori associated ulcer

Action

Stimulates the absorption of fluids and electrolytes in the intestinal wall, reduction in hypermotility of the stomach, and binds to toxins.

Therapeutic Class

antidiarrheal, antiulcer

Pharmacologic Class

adsorbant

Nursing Considerations

- **contraindicated in aspirin hypersensitivity**
- increase risk for impaction with geriatric and pediatric patients
- monitor liver profile
- bismuth may interfere with radiologic exams

Bupropion

Name

bupropion

Trade Name

Wellbutrin

Indication

depression, smoking cessation, treat ADHD in adults

Action

not well understood, ↑ dopamenergic and noradrenergic transmission via reuptake

Therapeutic Class

Antidepressants, smoking deterrents

Pharmacologic Class

aminoketones

Nursing Considerations

- **may lead to seizures, suicidal thoughts**
- **do not administer if patient is taking MAOI**
- use caution with renal and liver impairment
- assess mental status
- instruct patient to avoid alcohol (may lead to hallucinations, seizures, anxiety)

Buspirone

Generic Name

buspirone

Trade Name

Buspar

Indication

management of anxiety

Action

relieves anxiety by binding to dopamine and serotonin receptors

Therapeutic Class

Antidepressants, smoking deterrents

Pharmacologic Class

aminoketones

Nursing Considerations

- **do not administer concurrently with MOAI or grapefruit juice**
- may lead to dizziness, drowsiness, fatigue, and weakness
- patient may experience chest pain, palpitations, tachycardia
- instruct patient to take as directed
- instruct patient to avoid alcohol and other CNS depressants

Butorphanol

Generic Name

butorphanol

Trade Name

Stadol

Indication

moderate to severe pain, labor pain, sedation

Action

alters perception and response to pain by biding to opiate receptors in CNS

Therapeutic Class

Opioid Analgesic

Pharmacologic Class

opioid agonists/antagonists

Nursing Considerations

- use caution with concurrent use of MAOIs
- may cause confusion, hallucinations, sedation
- monitor for CNS depression
- **assess blood pressure pulse and respirations during administration**
- administer slowly through IV line

Calcium acetate

Generic Name

calcium acetate

Trade Name

PhosLo

Indication

treatment of hypocalcemia, prevention of post menopausal osteoporosis, treatment of hyperkalemia and hypermagnesaemia, adjunct in cardiac arrest, control of hyperphosphatemia with ESRD. Binds to phosphate in food and prevents absorption.

Action

calcium is essential for nervous muscular and skeletal systems, helps maintain cell membranes, aids in transmission of nerve impulses and muscle contraction, aids in blood formation and coagulation

Therapeutic Class

mineral and electrolyte replacements/supplements

Pharmacologic Class

antacids

Nursing Considerations

- **may cause cardiac arrest and arrhythmias**
- **phlebitis at site of insertion**
- monitor hemodynamics
- may cause hypotension, bradycardia, and arrhythmias
- hypercalcemia can increase risk for digoxin toxicity
- administer slowly
- instruct pt on foods that contain Vitamin D and encourage adequate intake.
- monitor parathyroid hormone

Calcium carbonate

Generic Name

calcium carbonate

Trade Name

Tums / Rolaids

Indication

treatment of hypocalcemia, prevention of post menopausal osteoporosis, treatment of hyperkalemia and hypermagnesaemia, used as antacid

Action

calcium is essential for nervous, muscular, and skeletal systems, helps maintain cell membranes, aids in transmission of nerve impulses and muscle contraction, aids in blood formation and coagulation

Therapeutic Class

mineral and electrolyte replacements/supplements

Pharmacologic Class

antacids

Nursing Considerations

- **may cause cardiac arrest and arrhythmias**
- monitor hemodynamics
- may causes hypotension, bradycardia, and arrhythmias
- **hypercalcemia can increase risk for digoxin toxicity**
- instruct pt on foods that contain Vitamin D and encourage adequate intake
- monitor parathyroid hormone

Captopril

Generic Name

captopril

Trade Name

Capoten

Indication

hypertension, management of CHF, decrease progression of DM neuropathy

Action

block conversion of angiotensin I to angiotensin II, increases renin levels and decreases aldosterone leading to vasodilation

Therapeutic Class

antihypertensives

Pharmacologic Class

ACE Inhibitor

Nursing Considerations

- can cause neutropenia - check WBCs regularly
- use cautiously with potassium supplements and potassium sparing diuretics
- use cautiously with diuretic therapy
- administer 1 hour before meals
- monitor blood pressure often
- monitor weight and fluid status
- monitor renal profile
- monitor CBC frequently
- may lead to Rhabdomyolysis
- **dry cough**

Carbamazepine

Generic Name

carbamazepine

Trade Name

Tegretol

Indication
seizures, DM neuropathy, pain associated with trigeminal neuralgia

Action

affects Na channels in neurons leading to decreased synaptic transmission

Therapeutic Class

Anticonvulsant

Pharmacologic Class

Nursing Considerations

- **interferes with oral contraceptives**
- do not use with MAOIs
- may cause suicidal thoughts
- may cause Stevens-Johnson syndrome, agranulocytosis, aplastic anemia, thrombocytopenia
- do not consume grapefruit juice while taking this medication
- monitor CBC and platelet count
- monitor serum blood levels of medication often

Carbidopa/levodopa

Generic Name

carbidopa/levodopa

Trade Name

Sinemet

Indication

Parkinson's disease

Action

levodopa is converted to dopamine and works as a neurotransmitter, carbidopa prevents the destruction of levodopa allowing it to cross the blood brain barrier

Therapeutic Class

Antiparkinson agent

Pharmacologic Class

Dopamine Agonist

Nursing Considerations

- may cause orthostatic hypotension
- **may cause dark urine**
- weeks to months to take effect
- do not use with MAOIs
- **do not use with glaucoma, melanoma**
- **assess for parkinsonian symptoms**
- instruct patient to take as directed

Cefaclor

Generic Name

cefaclor

Trade Name

Ceclor

Indication

treatment of respiratory tract infections, skin infections, otitis media

Action

bacteriacidal, binds to bacterial cell wall causing cell death

Therapeutic Class

anti-infectives

Pharmacologic Class

Cephalosporin 2nd generations

Nursing Considerations

- contraindicated in cephalosporin and possibly penicillin allergies
- may need lead to seizures, pseudomembranous colitis, diarrhea, phlebitis at IV site, anaphylaxis
- assess infection and allergies
- **obtain cultures prior to therapy**
- monitor bowel function
- may lead to super infection

Cefdinir

Generic Name

cefdinir

Trade Name

Omnicef

Indication

treatment of skin infections, otitis media

Action

bactericidal, binds to bacterial cell wall causing cell death

Therapeutic Class

anti-infectives

Pharmacologic Class

Cephalosporin 2nd generations

Nursing Considerations

- contraindicated in cephalosporin and possibly penicillin allergies
- may need lead to seizures, pseudomembranous colitis, diarrhea, phlebitis at IV site, anaphylaxis
- Assess infection and allergies
- obtain cultures prior to therapy
- monitor bowel function
- monitor for bleeding
- may lead to super infection

Celecoxib

Generic Name

celecoxib

Trade Name

Celebrex

Indication

osteoarthritis, rheumatoid arthritis, acute pain

Action

decreases pain and inflammation by inhibiting synthesis of prostaglandins

Therapeutic Class

antirrheumatics/NSAID

Pharmacologic Class

Nursing Considerations

- use caution with cardiovascular disease
- increases risk for MI, CVA, thrombosis
- **may cause GI bleeding, Stevens-Johnson syndrome, dermatitis**
- notify provider for new-onset abdominal pain or black stool

Cephalexin

Generic Name

cephalexin

Trade Name

Keflex

Indication

skin infections, pneumonia, UTI, otitis media

Action

bactericidal: binds to bacterial cell wall leading to cell death

Therapeutic Class

anti-infectives

Pharmacologic Class

Cephalosporin 1st generations

Nursing Considerations

* contraindicated with cephalosporin and serious penicillin allergies.
* may need lead to seizures, pseudomembranous colitis, diarrhea, phlebitis at IV site, anaphylaxis
* Assess infection and allergies
* obtain cultures prior to therapy
* monitor bowel function
* may lead to super infection
* may cause elevated liver enzymes

Chlorpromazine

Generic Name

chlorpromazine

Trade Name

Thorazine

Indication

second line treatment of schizophrenia and psychosis, nausea/vomiting, pre-op sedation, acute intermittent porphyria, headache, bipolar

Action

exhibits anticholinergic activity, alters effects of dopamine in CNS

Therapeutic Class

Antipsychotic, antiemetic

Pharmacologic Class

phenothiazines (dopamine D2 receptor antagonist)

Nursing Considerations

- may cause neuroliptic malignant syndrome, sedation, tardive dyskineisa, hypotenstion, agranulocytosis
- assess mental status prior to and during treatment
- monitor blood pressure
- ensure patient is taking medication
- monitor CBC and liver function tests
- instruct patient not to skip doses or double dose.

Cimetidine

Generic Name

cimetidine

Trade Name

Tagamet

Indication

treatment of duodenal ulcers, GERD, heartburn, Zollinger Ellison syndrome, prevention of GI bleeding in critical patients.

Action

inhibits action of histamine leading to inhibition of gastric acid secretion

Therapeutic Class

antiulcer agent

Pharmacologic Class

Histamine H2 antagonist

Nursing Considerations

- increases serum level of warfarin
- can lead to respiratory infection (green sputum)
- monitor for arryhtmias
- may cause agranulocytosis, aplastic anemia
- monitor CBC during therapy
- take medication as directed
- instruct patient to increase fluid and fiber intake to decrease constipation

Ciprofloxacin

Generic Name

ciprofloxacin

Trade Name

Cipro

Indication

urinary tract infections, gonorrhea, respiratory tract infections, bronchitis, pneumonia, skin and bone infections, infectious diarrhea, abdominal infections

Action

inhibits bacterial DNA synthesis

Therapeutic Class

anti-infectives

Pharmacologic Class

Fluoroquinolone

Nursing Considerations

- contraindicated in allergies
- **may cause QT prolongation**, avoid use with other drugs that can cause QT prolongation
- can cause seizures, arrythmias, pseudomembranous colitis, anaphalaxis, Stevens Johnson syndrome
- may decrease effects of phenytoin
- monitor renal panel
- assess for infection, obtain cultures prior to therapy
- monitor liver function tests

Clindamycin

Generic Name

clindamycin

Trade Name

Cleocin

Indication

skin infections, respiratory tract infections, septicemia, intra-abdominal infections, osteomyelitis

Action

bacteriostatic: inhibits protein synthesis

Therapeutic Class

Anti-infectives

Pharmacologic Class

Nursing Considerations

* arrythmias, pseudomembranous colitis, diarrhea, phlebitis
* monitor bowel function
* assess for infection, obtain cultures prior to therapy
* monitor liver function tests
* monitor CBC

Clopidogrel

Generic Name

clopidogrel

Trade Name

Plavix

Indication

atherosclerotic events, MI, CVA, PVD, acute coronary syndrome

Action

inhibits platelet aggregation

Therapeutic Class

Antiplatelet agent

Pharmacologic Class

platelet aggregation inhibitors

Nursing Considerations

- may cause GI bleeding, neutropenia, hypercholesterolemia
- may increase risk for bleeding in warfarin, aspirin, heparin
- can increase risk for bleeding with garlic, ginkgo, ginger
- monitor for signs of bleeding
- monitor bleeding times
- **monitor CBC and platelet count**
- **discontinue use 5-7 days before surgery**

Codeine

Generic Name

codeine

Trade Name

Paveral

Indication

management of pain, diarrhea, cough suppressant

Action

binds to opiate receptors in the CNS and alters perception of pain while producing a general depression of the CNS. This depression also causes a decrease in the cough reflex and GI motility.

Therapeutic Class

allergy, cold, cough remedy, antitussive, opioid analgesic

Pharmacologic Class

opioid agonist

Nursing Considerations

- may cause alterations in mentation, hypotension, constipation, nausea, vomiting
- **assess BP, pulse, and respiratory rate prior to administration and frequently during administration**
- use caution if patient is receiving MAO Inhibitors
- **Narcan (naloxone) is the antidote for opioid agonists**

Cortisone

Generic Name

cortisone

Trade Name

Cortone

Indication

management of adrenocortical insufficiency (Addison's Disease). Replace cortisol in states of deficiency, suppress inflammation and normal immune response.

Action

The adrenal glands sit on top of the kidneys.

The adrenal glands excrete steroid hormones, including cortisol that play a role in increasing blood sugars, immune suppression, and metabolism of fat, protein, and carbohydrates, as well as decreasing bone formation.

Therapeutic Class

antiasthmatics, corticosteroids

Pharmacologic Class

corticosteroids

Nursing Considerations

- Excreted by the liver - monitor liver profile
- Avoid in active untreated infections
- may cause CNS alterations
- may cause Cushingoid appearance (buffalo hump, moon face)
- Weight gain
- Osteoporosis
- Decrease wound healing

- May elevate blood sugars
- May increase cholesterol and lipid values

Cyclosporine

Generic Name

cyclosporine

Trade Name

Sandimmune

Indication

prevention of rejection in transplantation, treatment of severe RA, management of ulcerative colitis

Action

inhibits normal immune response primarily by decreasing the activity of T cells

Therapeutic Class

immunosuppressant, antirheumatics (DMARD)

Pharmacologic Class

polypeptides (cyclic)

Nursing Considerations

- **may cause seizures**, tremors, hypertension, hepatotoxicity, diarrhea, N/V, gingival hyperplasia
- **increases immune suppression with corticosteroids**
- avoid grapefruit juice while taking this medications
- assess for signs of organ rejection
- monitor renal panel, liver enzymes
- take medication as directed
- lifelong therapy required for transplant patients
- instruct pt on how to take blood pressure

Dexamethasone

Generic Name

dexamethasone

Trade Name

Decadron

Indication

manage cerebral edema, assess for Cushing's Disease

Action

Suppress inflammation and normal immune response. Used in inflammatory states to decrease inflammation.

Therapeutic Class

antiasthmatics, corticosteroids

Pharmacologic Class

corticosteroids

Nursing Considerations

- excreted by the liver - monitor liver profile
- avoid in active untreated infections
- may cause CNS alterations
- may cause peptic ulcers
- may cause Cushingoid appearance (buffalo hump, moon face)
- weight gain
- osteoporosis
- decrease wound healing
- may elevate blood sugars
- may increase cholesterol and lipid values

Diazepam

Generic Name

diazepam

Trade Name

Valium

Indication

anxiety, pre-op sedation, conscious sedation, treatment of seizures, insomnia, management of alcohol withdrawal

Action

decreases the effects of voltage gated sodium channels to depresses the CNS

Therapeutic Class

antianxiety agents, anticonvulsants, sedative/hypnotics, skeletal muscle relaxants (centrally acting)

Pharmacologic Class

Benzodiazepine

Nursing Considerations

- contraindicated in hepatic dysfunction
- use caution with renal impairment
- can cause dizziness, drowsiness, lethargy, hypotension, physical dependence, tolerance
- instruct patient to take as directed
- caution to avoid alcohol use
- Flumazenil (Romazicon) is the reversal agent

Digoxin

Generic Name

digoxin

Trade Name

Lanoxin

Indication

CHF, A-fib, A-flutter

Action

Positive inotropic effect (increases force of myocardial contraction), prolongs refractory period, ↓ conduction through SA and AV nodes. Essentially digoxin is given to increase cardiac output and slow the rate.

Therapeutic Class

antiarrhythmic, inotropics

Pharmacologic Class

digitalis glycosides

Nursing Considerations

- Excreted by kidneys
- Assess patient for hypersensitivity
- Contraindicated with uncontrolled ventricular arryhtmias
- Hypokalemia increase risk for toxicity
- Hypercalcemia ↑ risk for toxicity
- Use caution with diuretic use as they may cause electrolyte abnormalities that can lead to toxicity
- Assess patient for cardiac arrythmias including bradycardia
- Signs of toxicity include vision changes (blurred vision, yellow, green vision disturbances)

- Monitor pulse rate for 1 full minute prior to dosing patient (hold for pulse <60)

Diltiazem

Generic Name

diltiazem

Trade Name

Cardizem

Indication

hypertension, angina, SVT, a-fib, aflutter

Action

inhibits calcium transport resulting in inhibition of excitation and contraction, leads to depression of AV and SA node leading to decreased HR, leads to vasodilatation and decreased blood pressure.

Therapeutic Class

antianginals, antiarrhythmics, antihypertensive

Pharmacologic Class

Ca Channel Blocker (Bezothiazepine)

Nursing Considerations

- contraindicated in 2nd and 3rd AV block
- may cause arrhythmias, CHF, bradycardia, peripheral edema, gingival hyperplasia
- increases digoxin levels
- don't drink grapefruit juice
- assess for signs of CHF
- monitor EKG continuously
- tell patient to change positions slowly
- monitor serum potassium
- instruct pt on how to take blood pressure

Diphenhydramine

Generic Name

diphenhydramine

Trade Name

Benadryl

Indication

allergy, anaphylaxis, sedation, motion sickness, antitussive

Action

antagonizes effects of histamine, CNS depression

Therapeutic Class

allergy, cold and cough remedy, antihistamine, antitussive

Pharmacologic Class

Nursing Considerations

- **may cause drowsiness, anorexia, dry mouth, nausea, chest tightness, thick secretions, hypotension, blurred vision, headache**
- anticholinergic effects (dry mouth, blurred vision, constipation, sedation)
- assess purpose of medication prior to giving it
- assess allergies, sleep patterns, cough and lung sounds
- patient should avoid other over-the-counter cough and cold remedies

Diphenoxylate/Atropine

Generic Name

diphenoxylate/atropine

Trade Name

Lomotil

Indication

Treatment for diarrhea

Action

Inhibits GI motility via anticholinergic effects

Therapeutic Class

antidiarrheal

Pharmacologic Class

anticholinergic

Nursing Considerations

- contraindicated with angle-closure glaucoma, dehydration
- structurally related to opioids so use caution with patients that have allergies to opioids
- may cause constipation, tachycardia, dizziness, ileus
- monitor liver function as medication is excreted by the liver
- insure that client is taking medication as prescribed and not double dosing

Divalproex (valproic acid derivative)

Generic Name

divalproex

Trade Name

Depakote

Indication

seizures, manic episodes, prevention of headache

Action

increases the level of GABA (inhibitory neurotransmitter) in CNS

Therapeutic Class

Anticonvulsant, vascular headache suppressants

Pharmacologic Class

Nursing Considerations

- may cause suicidal thoughts, agitation, dizziness, insomnia, hepatotoxicity, pancreatitis
- increases risk for bleeding with Warfarin
- use caution with MAOIs
- monitor liver function tests

Dobutamine

Generic Name

dobutamine

Trade Name

Dobutrex

Indication

short term management of heart failure

Action

Dobutamine has a positive inotropic effect (increases cardiac output) with very little effect on heart rate. Stimulates $Beta_1$ receptors in the heart.

Therapeutic Class

inotropic

Pharmacologic Class

beta-adrenergic agonist

Nursing Considerations

- Monitor hemodynamics: hypertension, ↑HR, PVCs
- Skin reactions may occur with hypersensitivity
- Beta blockers may negate therapeutic effects of dobutamine
- Monitor cardiac output
- Monitor peripheral pulses before, during, and after therapy
- DO NOT confuse dobutamine with dopamine

Dopamine

Generic Name

dopamine

Trade Name

Intropin

Indication

used to improve blood pressure, cardiac output, and urine output

Action

Smaller doses result in renal vasodilation

Doses 2-10mcg/kg/min result in cardiac stimulation by acting on beta1 receptors

Doses >10mcg/kg/min stimulate alpha receptors leading to vasoconstriction (↑SVR)

Therapeutic Class

inotropic, vasopressor

Pharmacologic Class

adrenergic

Nursing Considerations

- Monitor hemodynamics closely: BP, HR, EKG, CVP, and PAOP if available
- Obtain parameters for hemodynamic values
- Titrate to obtain appropriate BP (more potent vasoconstrictors may be required)
- Irritation may occur at IV site
- Beta blockers may counteract therapeutic effects

Enalapril

Generic Name

enalapril

Trade Name

Vasotec

Indication
hypertension, management of CHF

Action

block conversion of angiotensin I to angiotensin II, increases renin levels and decreases aldosterone leading to vasodilation

Therapeutic Class

antihypertensives

Pharmacologic Class

ACE Inhibitor

Nursing Considerations

- can cause neutropenia - check WBCs regularly
- use cautiously with potassium supplements and potassium sparing diuretics.
- use cautiously with diuretic therapy
- administer 1 hour before meals
- monitor blood pressure often
- monitor weight and fluid status
- monitor renal profile
- monitor CBC frequently
- dry cough

Enoxaparin

Generic Name

enoxaparin

Trade Name

Lovenox

Indication

prevention of VTE, DVT, and PE

Action

prevents thrombus formation by potentiating the inhibitory effect of antithrombin on factor Xa and thrombin. Enoxaparin is a low molecular weight heparin.

Therapeutic Class

anticoagulant

Pharmacologic Class

antithrombotic

Nursing Considerations

- contraindicated in pork hypersensitivity
- monitor for signs of bleeding
- administer in subcutaneous tissue
- **DO NOT eject air bubble prior to injection**
- **DO NOT aspirate or massage site**

Epinephrine

Generic Name

epinephrine

Trade Name

Adrenalin, EpiPen

Indication

asthma and COPD exacerbations, allergic reactions, cardiac arrest, anesthesia adjunct

Action

Affects both beta$_1$ and beta$_2$ also has alpha agonist properties resulting in bronchodilation and increases in HR and BP. Inhibits hypersensitivity reactions.

Therapeutic Class

antiasthmatic, bronchodilator, vasopressor

Pharmacologic Class

adrenergic agonist

Nursing Considerations

- Side effects include: angina, tachycardia, hypertension, restlessness, nervousness, hyperglycemia
- Use with MAOI may lead to hypertensive crisis
- Patients should not use stimulants (caffeine, guarana, etc)
- Excessive use may cause bronchospasm
- Assess lung sounds, pulse, BP, and other hemodynamic parameters
- Monitor for chest pain
- Instruct patient to use as directed
- Patient should insure adequate fluid intake to liquefy secretions
- Mouth should be rinsed after inhalation
- Beta blockers may negate effects
- May increase blood glucose levels

Epoetin

Generic Name

epoetin

Trade Name

Epogen

Indication

anemia

Action

stimulates erythropoesis (production of RBCs)

Therapeutic Class

antianemics

Pharmacologic Class

hormones

Nursing Considerations

- contraindicated in albumin hypersensitivity
- may cause seizures, CHF, MI, CVA, HTN
- monitor blood pressure during therapy
- monitor for signs of anemia
- **assess dialysis shunts**
- monitor bleeding times
- initiate seizure precautions
- do not shake vial
- more information on Erythropoiesis
  (http://en.wikipedia.org/wiki/Erythropoiesis)

Erythromycin

Generic Name

erythromycin

Trade Name

E-Mycin

Indication

useful in place of penicillin when patient cannot take penicillin, upper and lower respiratory tract infections, otitis media, skin infections, pertussis, syphilis, rheumatic fever

Action

Bacteriostatic: suppresses bacterial protein synthesis

Therapeutic Class

anti-infective

Pharmacologic Class

macrolide

Nursing Considerations

- Causes **QT prolongation**, ventricular arrhythmias
- diarrhea
- asses infection
- monitor liver function tests
- instruct patient to finish medication dosage even if they are feeling better
- medication should not be shared

Escitalopram

Generic Name

escitalopram

Trade Name

Lexapro

Indication

major depressive disorder, anxiety disorder, PCD, PTSD, social phobia

Action

Increases the extracellular levels of serotonin in the synaptic cleft by selectively inhibiting its reuptake

Therapeutic Class

Antidepressant

Pharmacologic Class

SSRI

Nursing Considerations

- contraindicated with MAOI
- may cause suicidal thoughts, insomnia, drowsiness, diarrhea, nausea, serotonin syndrome
- may cause QT prolongation with certain medications
- assess for sexual dysfunction
- may take 4-6 weeks for full affect to take place
- monitor for serotonin syndrome (mental changes, NV, tachycardia, hyperthermia)

Famotidine

Generic Name

famotidine

Trade Name

Pepcid

Indication

short term treatment of active ulcer, GERD, treatment of heartburn, indigestion, management of Zollinger Ellison syndrome, prevention of GI bleeding in critically ill patients, management of symptoms associated with overuse of NSAIDs

Action

blocks action of histamine located in gastric parietal cells, inhibits gastric acid secretion

Therapeutic Class

antiulcer agent

Pharmacologic Class

Histamine H2 antagonist

Nursing Considerations

- may cause arrythmias, agranulocytosis, aplastic anemias
- assess for abdominal pain and occult blood
- monitor CBC
- instruct pt to increase fluid and fiber intake to prevent constipation

Fentanyl

Generic Name

fentanyl

Trade Name

Sublimaze

Indication

supplement to general anesthesia, continuous IV infusion for purpose of analgesia

Action

binds to opiate receptors in CNS altering perception of pain, producing CNS depression

Therapeutic Class

Opioid Analgesic

Pharmacologic Class

opioid agonists

Nursing Considerations

- use caution with increased ICP, head trauma, adrenal insufficiency
- avoid use with MAOIs
- may cause apnea, laryngospasm, decreased respirations, bradycardia, hypotension
- do not consume grapefruit while taking this medication
- monitor hemodynamics during administration
- assess patient pain scale frequently

Ferrous Sulfate

Generic Name

ferrous sulfate

Trade Name

Feosol

Indication

prevention and treatment of iron-deficiency anemia

Action

Iron is essential for hemoglobin, myoglobin and enzymes, it is transported to organs where it becomes part of iron stores

Therapeutic Class

antianemics

Pharmacologic Class

iron supplements

Nursing Considerations

- may cause seizures, hypotension, constipation, epigastric pain, diarrhea, skin staining, anaphylaxis
- assess nutritional status, bowel function
- monitor hemoglobin, hematocrit, iron levels
- may cause elevated liver enzymes
- take on an empty stomach to increase absorption/vitamin c helps with absorption
- use z-track for IM injections

Fluoxetine

Generic Name

fluoxetine

Trade Name

Prozac

Indication

depressive disorder, OCD, bulimia, panic disorder, bipolar, anorexia, ADHD, DM neuropathy, obesity

Action

inhibits reuptake of serotonin allowing it to persist longer in the synaptic cleft

Therapeutic Class

Antidepressant

Pharmacologic Class

SSRI

Nursing Considerations

- do not use while taking MAOIs
- may cause suicidal thoughts, drowsiness, anxiety, sexual dysfunction, insomnia, palpitations
- monitor closely for serotonin syndrome
- concurrent use with certain medications may lead to QT prolongation
- monitor mood changes and assess for suicidal ideation
- monitor nutrition status
- may cause elevated liver enzymes
- instruct pt to maintain good oral hygiene

Fluticasone

Generic Name

Fluticasone

Trade Name

Flovent

Indication

prophylactic asthma treatment

Action

locally acting anti-inflammatory

Therapeutic Class

antiasthmatics, anti-inflammatory (steroid)

Pharmacologic Class

Coticosteroids, Inhalation

Nursing Considerations

- use cautiously with untreated infections and suppressed immune function
- may cause headache, insomnia, bronchospasm, nasal congestion, adrenal suppression
- monitor patient's respiratory status
- may lead to decreased bone density
- instruct patients using corticosteroids and bronchodilators that they need to use bronchodilators first.
- instruct patient to stop smoking

Furosemide

Generic Name

Furosemide

Trade Name

Lasix

Indication

edema, hypertension

Action

prevents reabsorption of sodium and chloride in the kidneys, increase excretion of water, sodium, chloride, magnesium, potassium

Therapeutic Class

diuretics

Pharmacologic Class

loop diuretics

Nursing Considerations

- use caution with liver disease
- may cause hypotension, dry mouth, excessive urination, dehydration, electrolyte abnormalities, metabolic alkalosis
- **hypokalemia may lead to increase risk of digoxin toxicity**
- monitor renal panel
- use caution with other anithypertensives
- causes arthritic symptoms/do not administer with aminoglycosides due to ototoxicity

Gabapentine

Generic Name

gabapentine

Trade Name

Neurontin

Indication

seizures, peripheral neuropathy, neuropathic pain, prevention of migraines

Action

exact method of action unknown, may play a role in stabilizing neural membranes

Therapeutic Class

analgesic adjuncts, therapeutic, anticonvulsants, mood stabilizers

Pharmacologic Class

Nursing Considerations

- may cause suicidal thoughts, confusion, depression, drowsiness, ataxia, facial edema, hypertension
- monitor pt closely for changes in behavior and depression
- assess seizure activity
- assess pain level
- patient should take medications exactly as prescribed

Gentamicin

Generic Name

gentamicin

Trade Name

Cidomycin

Indication

Treatment of gram negative infections when penicillin is ineffective

Action

Inhibits bacterial protein synthesis

Therapeutic Class

anti-infectives

Pharmacologic Class

Aminoglycoside

Nursing Considerations

- causes tinnitus-hearing loss/do not administer with penicillin
- use caution in renal impairment
- assess for infection
- obtain cultures prior to therapy
- monitor liver function tests
- monitor blood levels of drug

Glipizide

Generic Name

glipizide

Trade Name

Glucotrol

Indication

type 2 diabetes mellitus

Action

stimulates release of insulin from the beta cells in the pancreases and leads to increased sensitivity to insulin

Therapeutic Class

anti-diabetic

Pharmacologic Class

sulfonylureas

Nursing Considerations

- may cause aplastic anemias, hypoglycemia, photosensitivity, dizziness, drowsiness, headache, diarrhea
- monitor CBC, assess for allergy to sulfonamides
- beta blockers may create signs of hypoglycemia
- instruct patient on how to check blood sugars and
- instruct patient on importance of carrying source of sugar in case of hypoglycemia

Glucagon

Generic Name

glucagon

Trade Name

GlucaGen

Indication

severe hypoglycemia, antidote for beta blockers and calcium channel blockers

Action

stimulates production of glucose from stores, relaxes GI tract

Therapeutic Class

hormones

Pharmacologic Class

pancreatics

Nursing Considerations

- may cause anaphylaxis
- may cause hypotension
- assess for signs of hypoglycemia, neuro status
- monitor serum glucose levels
- teach patient signs of hypoglycemia

Guaifenesin

Generic Name

guaifenesin

Trade Name

Robitussin

Indication

Cough suppression, expectorant

Action

Decreases viscosity of and mobilizes secretions

Therapeutic Class

allergy, cold and cough remedies, expectorant

Pharmacologic Class

Nursing Considerations

- patient should avoid over the counter cold medications
- assess lung sounds
- maintain adequate fluid intake

Haloperidol

Generic Name

haloperidol

Trade Name

Haldol

Indication

Schizophrenia, mania, aggressive and agitated patient

Action

Alters the effect of dopamine

Therapeutic Class

Antipsychotic

Pharmacologic Class

butyrophenones

Nursing Considerations

- extrapyramidal symptoms, tardive dyskinesia
- use caution in QT prolongation
- may cause seizures, constipation, dry mouth, agranulosytosis
- assess for hallucinations
- monitor hemodynamics
- monitor for neuroleptic malignant syndrome (fever, muscular rigidity, altered mental status, and autonomic dysfunction)
- monitor CBC with differential

Heparin

Generic Name

heparin

Trade Name

Hep-Lock

Indication

Venous thromboembolism prophylaxis and treatment, low dose used to ensure patency of IV catheters

Action

increases the inhibitory effect of antithrombin on factor Xa

Therapeutic Class

anticoagulant

Pharmacologic Class

antithrombotic

Nursing Considerations

- **monitor for signs of bleeding**
- monitor platelet count
- may cause hyperkalemia
- have patient report any signs of bleeding

Hydralazine

Generic Name

hydralazine

Trade Name

Apresoline

Indication

hypertension

Action

arterial vasodilation by unclarified mechanism

Therapeutic Class

anti-hypertensive

Pharmacologic Class

vasodilator

Nursing Considerations

- may cause tachycardia, sodium retention, arrhythmias, angina
- use caution with MAOIs
- **monitor blood pressure**
- instruct patient on how to take blood pressure

Hydrochlorothiazide

Generic Name

hydrochlorothiazide

Trade Name

HydroDiuril

Indication

Hypertension, CHF, renal dysfunction, cirrhosis, glucocorticoid therapy

Action

Increases sodium and water excretion and produces arterial vasodilation

Therapeutic Class

antihypertensives, diuretics

Pharmacologic Class

thiazide diuretics

Nursing Considerations

- May cause dizziness, hypokalemia, hyponatremia, hypophosphatemia, hypomagnesemia, dehydration
- Hypokalemia can increase risk for digoxin toxicity
- Monitor blood pressure and intake and output
- Monitor electrolyte levels
- Patient should take medication at the same time each day even if feeling better
- Instruct patient on how to take blood pressure

Hydrocodone/Acetaminophen

Generic Name

hydrocodone/acetaminophen

Trade Name

Norco

Indication

management of moderate to severe pain

Action

alters the perception and reaction to pain by binding to opiate receptors in the CNS, also suppresses the cough reflex

Therapeutic Class

opioid Analgesic, allergy, cold and cough remedies, antitussive

Pharmacologic Class

opioid agonists, nonopioid analgesic combinations

Nursing Considerations

- use caution with concurrent use of MAOI - avoid use within 14 days of each other
- hypotension - monitor hemodynamics and respirations after administering
- may increase ICP use caution with head trauma
- Narcan (nalaxone) is the antidote for overdose
- **DO NOT exceed 4g of acetaminophen per day**

Hydromorphone

Generic Name

hydromorphone

Trade Name

Dilaudid

Indication

moderate to severe pain

Action

alters the perception and reaction to pain by binding to opiate receptors in the CNS, also suppresses the cough reflex

Therapeutic Class

Opioid Analgesic, allergy, cold and cough remedies, antitussive

Pharmacologic Class

opioid agonist

Nursing Considerations

- Assess BP, respirations, and pulse before and during administration - medication causes general CNS depression
- Narcan (nalaxone) is the antidote for overdose
- use caution with concurrent use of MAOI - avoid use within 14 days of each other
- may be used as an antitussive
- advised to dilute with NS prior to administration and to administer slowly to decrease CNS depression

Ibuprofen

Generic Name

ibuprofen

Trade Name

Advil / Motrin

Indication

Mild to moderate pain, inflammatory states

Action

Decreases pain and inflammation by inhibiting prostaglandins

Therapeutic Class

antipyretics, antirheumatics, nonopioid analgesics, nonsteroidal anti-inflammatory agents

Pharmacologic Class

nonopioid analgesics

Nursing Considerations

- may cause GI bleeding, hepatitis, Stevens-Johnson Syndrome
- may cause anaphylaxis
- monitor for headache, nausea, vomiting, constipation
- therapy should be discontinued after first sign of rash
- monitor renal and liver labs
- patient should avoid using alcohol

Indomethacin

Generic Name

indomethacin

Trade Name

Indocin

Indication

Inflammatory disorders when patients do not respond to other medications

Action

Decreases pain and inflammation by inhibiting prostaglandin synthesis

Therapeutic Class

antirheumatics, ductus arteriosus patency adjuncts (IV only), nonsteroidal anti-inflammatory agents

Pharmacologic Class

Nursing Considerations

- monitor for hepatitis and GI bleeding
- monitor for dizziness, drowsiness, and headache
- assess for anaphylactic reaction
- aspirin may decrease effectiveness
- monitor renal labs
- shake suspension before administration
- patient should wear sunscreen and protective clothing to protect against photosensitivity

Insulin- short acting

Generic Name

regular

Trade Name

Humulin R/Novolin R

Indication

hyperglycemia with diabetes type 1 and 2, diabetic ketoacidosis

Action

stimulates uptake of glucose into muscle and fat cells, inhibits production of glucose in the liver, prevents breakdown of fat and protein

Route	Onset	Peak	Duration
Subcutaneous	30-45 min	1.5-2.5h	4.5-6h

Therapeutic Class

antidiabetics, hormones

Pharmacologic Class

pancreatics

Nursing Considerations

- assess for symptoms of hypoglycemia or hyperglycemia
- monitor body weight over time
- may cause decreased inorganic phosphates, potassium, and magnesium
- monitor blood sugars every 6 hours, monitor A1C every 3-6 months

Insulin- intermediate acting

Generic Name

NPH

Trade Name

Humulin N, Novolin N

Indication

hyperglycemia with diabetes type 1 and 2, diabetic ketoacidosis

Action

stimulates uptake of glucose into muscle and fat cells, inhibits production of glucose in the liver, prevents breakdown of fat and protein

Route	Onset	Peak	Duration
Subcutaneous	1-2 hr	4-12hr	18-24hr

Therapeutic Class

antidiabetics, hormones

Pharmacologic Class

pancreatics

Nursing Considerations

- assess for symptoms of hypoglycemia or hyperglycemia
- monitor body weight over time
- may cause decreased inorganic phosphates, potassium, and magnesium
- monitor blood sugars every 6 hours, monitor A1C every 3-6 months

Insulin- long acting

Generic Name

detemir, glargine

Trade Name

Levemir, Lantus

Indication

hyperglycemia with diabetes type 1 and 2, diabetic ketoacidosis

Action

stimulates uptake of glucose into muscle and fat cells, inhibits production of glucose in the liver, prevents breakdown of fat and protein

Route	Onset	Peak	Duration
Detemir	3-4 hr	3-14 hr	24 hr
Glargine	3-4 hr	none	24 hr

Therapeutic Class

antidiabetics, hormones

Pharmacologic Class

pancreatics

Nursing Considerations

- assess for symptoms of hypoglycemia or hyperglycemia
- monitor body weight over time
- may cause decreased inorganic phosphates, potassium, and magnesium
- monitor blood sugars every 6 hours, monitor A1C every 3-6 months

Insulin- rapid acting

Generic Name

aspart, lispro, glulisine

Trade Name

novolog, humalog, apidra

Indication

hyperglycemia with diabetes type 1 and 2, diabetic ketoacidosis

Action

stimulates uptake of glucose into muscle and fat cells, inhibits production of glucose in the liver, prevents breakdown of fat and protein

Route	Onset	Peak	Duration
Aspart	10-20 min	1-3 hr	3-5 hr
Glulisine	15 min	1 hr	2-4 hr
Lispro	15 min	1-1.5 hr	3-4 hr

Therapeutic Class

antidiabetics, hormones

Pharmacologic Class

pancreatics

Nursing Considerations

- assess for symptoms of hypoglycemia or hyperglycemia
- monitor body weight over time
- may cause decreased inorganic phosphates, potassium, and magnesium
- monitor blood sugars every 6 hours, monitor A1C every 3-6 months

Insulin-mixtures

Generic Name

Lispro mixture, Aspart mixture, NPH/regular

Trade Name

Humalog Mix, NovoLog Mix, Humulin 70/30, Novolin 70/30

Indication

hyperglycemia with diabetes type 1 and 2, diabetic ketoacidosis

Action

stimulates uptake of glucose into muscle and fat cells, inhibits production of glucose in the liver, prevents breakdown of fat and protein

Route	Onset	Peak	Duration
Lispro mix	15-30 min	2-3 hr	24 hr
Aspart mix	15 min	1-4 hr	18-24 hr
NPH regular	30 min	4-8 hr	24 hr

Therapeutic Class

antidiabetics, hormones

Pharmacologic Class

pancreatics

Nursing Considerations

- assess for symptoms of hypoglycemia or hyperglycemia
- monitor body weight over time
- may cause decreased inorganic phosphates, potassium, and magnesium
- monitor blood sugars every 6 hours, monitor A1C every 3-6 months

Iodine

Generic Name

radioactive iodine

Trade Name

Indication

thyroidectomy pretreatment, thyrotoxic crisis, radiation exposure

Action

inhibits the release of thyroid hormones

Therapeutic Class

Antithyroid Agent, control of hyperthyroidism

Pharmacologic Class

Nursing Considerations

- may cause GI bleeding, diarrhea, hypothyroidism, goiter
- monitor for hypersensitivity

Isoniazide

Generic Name

isoniazide

Trade Name

INH

Indication

tuberculosis

Action

Inhibits synthesis of mycobacterial cell wall

Therapeutic Class

Antitubercular

Pharmacologic Class

Nursing Considerations

- can cause jaundice
- may cause peripheral neuropathy, seizures, hepatitis
- patient should avoid high amounts of tyramine (pickled meats, aged/smoked meats, alcohol, exotic/aged cheese)
- monitor liver function tests
- complete full course of therapy (6-12 months)
- often used in combination with Rifampin

Ketorolac

Generic Name

ketorolac

Trade Name

Toradol

Indication

pain

Action

pain relief due to prostaglandin inhibition by blocking of the enzyme cyclooxygenase (COX)

Therapeutic Class

nonsteroidal anti-inflammatory agents, nonopioid analgesics

Pharmacologic Class

pyrroziline carboxylic acid

Nursing Considerations

- may cause GI bleeding, Stevens-Johnson Syndrome, anaphylaxis, drowsiness
- **should not exceed 5 days of therapy**
- bleeding risk increased with garlic, ginger, and ginkgo
- may decrease effectiveness of hypertensive medications and diuretics

Lactulose

Generic Name

lactulose

Trade Name

Kristalose

Indication

Constipation, portal-systemic encephalopathy

Action

draws water into the stool and softens stool, inhibits ammonia passing into the colon

Therapeutic Class

laxative

Pharmacologic Class

osmotic

Nursing Considerations

- use caution with DM
- may cause cramps, abdominal distention, hyperglycemia
- assess mental status, ammonia levels, abdominal distention
- patient should average 2-3 bowel movements per day

Lamotrigine

Generic Name

lamotrigine

Trade Name

Lamictal

Indication

seizures r/t epilepsy, bipolar

Action

Inhibits sodium transport in neurons

Therapeutic Class

anticonvulsant

Nursing Considerations

- may cause suicidal thoughts, dizziness, behavior changes, nausea, vomiting, photosensitivity, rash, Stevens-Johnson Syndrome
- use caution with oral contraceptive use
- assess mental status
- assess for seizures
- do not discontinue use abruptly

Levetiracetam

Generic Name

levetiracetam

Trade Name

Keppra

Indication

Seizures

Action

decreases severity and incidence of seizures by inhibiting presynaptic calcium channels and reducing neurotransmitter realease

Therapeutic Class

anticonvulsants

Pharmacologic Class

pyrrolidines

Nursing Considerations

- May cause suicidal thoughts, dizziness, weakness
- May alter RBC, WBC, and liver function
- May cause somnolence
- **Should be infused over 15 minutes**

Levofloxacin

Generic Name

levofloxacin

Trade Name

Levaquin

Indication

urinary tract infections, gonorrhea, respiratory tract infections, bronchitis, pneumonia, skin and bone infections

Action

inhibits DNA synthesis in bacteria

Therapeutic Class

Anti-infective

Pharmacologic Class

fluoroquinolone

Nursing Considerations

- contraindicated in allergies
- may cause **QT prolongation**, avoid use with other drugs that can cause QT prolongation
- can cause seizures, arrythmias, pseudomembranous colitis, anaphylaxis, Stevens Johnson syndrome
- may decreased of phenytoin
- monitor renal panel
- assess for infection, obtain cultures prior to therapy
- monitor liver function tests

Levothyroxine

Generic Name

levothyroxine

Trade Name

Levothroid

Indication

thyroid hormone replacement in hypothyroidism

Action

replaces thyroid hormone, increasing metabolism, promotes gluconeogenesis, stimulates protein synthesis, restores normal hormone balance and suppresses thyroid cancer

Therapeutic Class

hormone

Pharmacologic Class

thyroid preparations

Nursing Considerations

- assess pulse and monitor for **tachyarrythmias** and chest pain
- monitor TSH levels
- overdose is presented as hyperthyroidism
- start with low doses and increase as indicated
- **therapy is lifelong**
- take directly after breast feeding
- increases the effects of warfarin

Lisipnorpil

Generic Name

lisinopril

Trade Name

Prinivil

Indication

hypertension, management of CHF

Action

block conversion of angiotensin I to angiotensin II, increases renin levels and decreases aldosterone leading to vasodilation

Therapeutic Class

antihypertensives

Pharmacologic Class

ACE Inhibitor

Nursing Considerations

- **dry cough**
- **first dose hypotension**
- use cautiously with potassium supplements and potassium sparing diuretics.
- use cautiously with diuretic therapy
- administer 1 hour before meals
- monitor blood pressure often
- monitor weight and fluid status
- monitor renal profile
- monitor liver function tests

Lithium

Generic Name

lithium

Trade Name

Lithizine

Indication

mania

Action

alters cation transport and neurotransmitter reuptake

Therapeutic Class

Mood Stabilizer

Pharmacologic Class

Nursing Considerations

- do not administer with NSAIDs
- monitor drug blood levels frequently
- may cause seizures, arrhythmias, fatigue, confusion, nausea, anorexia, hypothyroidism, tremors
- Ace Inhibitors may increase serum levels
- instruct patient to maintain adequate fluid intake
- **therapeutic level: 0.5-1.5 mEq/L**

Loperamide

Generic Name

loperamide

Trade Name

Imodium

Indication

acute diarrhea, decrease drainage post ileostomy

Action

inhibits peristalsis, reduces the volume of feces while increasing the bulk and viscosity

Therapeutic Class

antidiarrheal

Nursing Considerations

- **may lead to constipation - insure proper use**
- assess bowel function
- assess fluid and electrolyte levels

Lorazepam

Generic Name

lorazepam

Trade Name

Ativan

Indication

anxiety, sedation, seizures

Action

general CNS depression by potentiating inhibitory neurotransmitters

Therapeutic Class

anesthetic adjuncts, antianxiety agents, sedative hypnotics

Pharmacologic Class

Benzodiazepine

Nursing Considerations

* use caution with COPD and sleep apnea
* avoid alcohol use
* antidote is Flumazenil (Romazicon)
* may cause apnea, cardiac arrest, bradycardia, hypotension
* use caution with other CNS depressants
* administer slowly and dilute to decrease complications

Losartan

Generic Name

losartan

Trade Name

Cozaar

Indication

hypertension, DM neuropathy, CHF

Action

inhibits vasoconstrictive properties of angiotensin II

Therapeutic Class

antihypertensives

Pharmacologic Class

angiotensin II receptor antagonist

Nursing Considerations

- may cause hypotension, tacycardia, angiodema, hyperkalemia
- may increase digoxin levels
- assess blood pressure and heart rate
- assess fluid levels
- monitor daily weights with CHF
- monitor renal and liver
- instruct patient on how to take blood pressure

Magnesium Sulfate

Generic Name

magnesium sulfate

Trade Name

MgSO4

Indication

treatment of hypomagnesaemia, hypertension, preterm labor, torsade de pointes, asthma, anticonvulsant with eclampsia

Action

magnesium plays a role in muscle excitability

Therapeutic Class

mineral and electrolyte replacements/supplements

Pharmacologic Class

minerals/electrolytes

Nursing Considerations

- use caution with renal insufficiency
- may cause decreased respiratory rate, arrythmias, hypotension, muscle weakness
- **monitor EKG and respiratory status**
- monitor Mg levels
- ensure dosage with secondary practitioner
- **Calcium gluconate is the antidote**
  - o Magnesium toxicity results in respiratory depress and loss of deep tendon reflexes

Mannitol

Generic Name

mannitol

Trade Name

Osmitrol

Indication

increased ICP, oliguric renal failure, edema, intraocular pressure

Action

inhibits reabsorption of water and electrolytes by increasing osmotic pressure, excreted by kidneys

Therapeutic Class

diuretic

Pharmacologic Class

osmotic diuretic

Nursing Considerations

- may cause phlebitis at IV site
- may cause dehydration, fluid and electrolyte imbalances
- monitor neuro status
- **administer via a filter**

Meperidine

Generic Name

meperidine

Trade Name

Demerol

Indication

moderate to severe pain, sedation

Action

Binds to opiate receptors in the CNS and alters perception of pain while producing a general depression of the CNS.

Therapeutic Class

Opioid Analgesic

Pharmacologic Class

opioid agonists

Nursing Considerations

- may cause alterations in mentation, hypotension, constipation, nausea, vomiting
- assess BP, pulse, and respiratory rate prior to administration and frequently during administration
- use caution if patient is receiving MAOIs
- Narcan (naloxone) is the antidote for opioid agonists
- can cause seizure
- may increase pancreatic enzyme levels
- assess bowel function

Metformin

Generic Name

metformin

Trade Name

Glucophage

Indication

management of Type II DM, PCOS

Action

decreases glucose production in the liver, decreases absorption, increases cellular insulin sensitivity

Therapeutic Class

Antidiabetic

Pharmacologic Class

Biguanide

Nursing Considerations

- do not use with renal dysfunction, metabolic acidosis
- may cause diarrhea, nausea, vomiting, lactic acidosis
- monitor patient closely for ketoacidosis and lactic acidosis, discontinue medication immediately if acidotic
- may cause metallic taste
- instruct patient that medication does not cure diabetes

Methadone

Generic Name

methadone

Trade Name

Mathadose

Indication

withdrawal symptoms, pain

Action

Suppresses withdrawal symptoms. Binds to opiate receptors in the CNS and alters perception of pain while producing a general depression of the CNS. This depression also causes a decrease in the cough reflex and GI motility.

Therapeutic Class

opioid analgesic

Pharmacologic Class

opioid agonist

Nursing Considerations

- use caution if patient is receiving MAO Inhibitors
- may cause **QT prolongation**, hypotension, respiratory depression, dependence, confusion, sedation
- assess pain, vital signs, bowel function
- may increase pancreatic enzyme levels
- assess withdrawal symptoms

Methylergonovine

Generic Name

methylergonovine

Trade Name

Methergine

Indication

treatment of post-partum hemorrhage

Action

stimulates uterine muscles causing uterine contraction

Therapeutic Class

oxytocic

Pharmacologic Class

ergot alkaloids

Nursing Considerations

- can cause hypertension, cramps, nausea, vomiting, dyspnea
- monitor BP, heart rate, uterine response
- **assess calcium levels** - effectiveness ↓ with hypocalcemia
- **monitor uterine bleeding** and notify physician of any changes

Methylphenidate

Generic Name

methylphenidate

Trade Name

Ritalin

Indication

ADHD, narcolepsy

Action

improves attention span in ADHD by producing CNS stimulation

Therapeutic Class

central nervous system stimulant

Pharmacologic Class

Nursing Considerations

- can cause sudden death, hypertension, palpitations, anorexia, hyperactivity, insomnia
- may decrease effects of Warfarin and Phenytoin
- do not use with MAOIs
- monitor cardiovascular system
- monitor for behavioral changes
- **monitor for dependence**
- **do not consume caffeinated beverages**

"**Drug Holiday**" used to assess dependence and status

Methylprednisone

Generic Name

methylprednisone

Trade Name

Solu-medrol

Indication

Inflammation, allergy, autoimmune disorders, prevent organ rejection

Action

Suppress inflammation and normal immune response. The adrenal glands excrete steroid hormones that play a role in increasing blood sugars, immune suppression, and metabolism of fat, protein, and carbohydrates, as well as decreasing bone formation.

Therapeutic Class

antiasthmatics, corticosteroids

Pharmacologic Class

corticosteroids

Nursing Considerations

- avoid in active untreated infections
- may cause CNS alterations
- may cause peptic ulcers
- may cause Cushingoid appearance (buffalo hump, moon face)
- weight gain
- osteoporosis
- decrease wound healing
- may elevate blood sugars
- may increase cholesterol and lipid values
- depress immune system/report signs of infection (sore throat)
- avoid grapefruit juice

Metoclopramide

Generic Name

metoclopramide

Trade Name

Reglan

Indication

prevention of nausea, vomiting, hiccups, migraines, gastric stasis

Action

accelerates gastric emptying by stimulating motility

Therapeutic Class

antiemetic

Pharmacologic Class

Nursing Considerations

- do not use with GI obstruction
- may cause extrapyramidal reaction, neurolyptic malignant syndrome, tardive dyskinesia, arrhythmias, blood pressure alterations, hematologic alterations, facial movements, sedation
- can decrease effects of levodopa
- assess nausea/vomiting
- monitor liver function tests

Metoprolol

Generic Name

metoprolol

Trade Name

Lopressor

Indication

tachyarrhythmias, HTN, angina, prevention of MI, heart failure management, may be used for migraine prophylaxis

Action

blocks the stimulation of beta$_1$ receptors in the SNS, does not usually effect on beta$_2$ receptors (cardioselective)

Therapeutic Class

antianginal, antihypertensive

Pharmacologic Class

beta blocker

Nursing Considerations

- **monitor hemodynamics**
- may lead to bradycardia, pulmonary edema
- use caution with MAOIs
- assess I&Os and monitor for signs of CHF

Metronidazole

Generic Name

metronidazole

Trade Name

Flagyl

Indication

intra-abdominal infections, gynecoligical infections, skin infections, bone and joint infections, CNS infections, septicemia, endocarditis, amebic liver abscess, peptic ulcer disease

Action

Inhibits DNA and protein synthesis in bacteria, bactericidal

Therapeutic Class

anti-infectives, antiprotozoals, antiulcer agents

Pharmacologic Class

Nursing Considerations

- do not take with alcohol-disulfiram reaction
- assess for infection before and during treatment
- **obtain cultures before therapy**
- monitor neurologic status: parasthesia, weakness, ataxia, or seizures
- monitor intake and output, daily weights
- may alter liver enzyme tests

Midazolam

Generic Name

midazolam

Trade Name

Versed

Indication

sedation, conscious sedation, anesthesia, status epilepticus

Action

acts to produce CNS depression, may be mediated by GABA

Therapeutic Class

antianxiety agent, sedative/hypnotics

Pharmacologic Class

Benzodiazepine

Nursing Considerations

- assess level of sedation during and for 2-6 hours following
- monitor blood pressure, pulse, respirations during IV administration
- may lead to apnea, cardiac arrest, respiratory depression
- antidote for overdose is Romazicon (flumazenil)

Montelukast

Generic Name

montelukast

Trade Name

Singulair

Indication

prevent or treat asthma, manage seasonal allergies, prevent exercise-induced bronchoconstriction

Action

disrupts the effects of leukotrienes which effect airway edema, smooth muscle constriction, and cellular activity

Therapeutic Class

allergy, cold, and cough remedies, bronchodilators

Pharmacologic Class

Leukotriene Antagonist

Nursing Considerations

- assess respiratory status
- assess liver function tests
- medication does not treat acute asthma attacks

Morphine

Generic Name

morphine

Trade Name

MS Contin

Indication

pain, pulmonary edema, MI

Action

Binds to opiate receptors in the CNS and alters perception of pain while producing a general depression of the CNS.

Therapeutic Class

opioid analgesic

Pharmacologic Class

opioid agonist

Nursing Considerations

- may cause alterations in mentation, hypotension, constipation, nausea, vomiting
- **assess BP, pulse, and respiratory rate prior to administration and frequently during administration**
- use caution if patient is receiving MAO Inhibitors
- **Narcan (naloxone)** is the antidote for opioid agonists

Nalbuphine

Generic Name

nalbuphine

Trade Name

Nubain

Indication

pain, analgesia during labor, sedation before surgery, supplement to balance anesthesia

Action

alters perception and response to pain, causes CNS depression

Therapeutic Class

Opioid Analgesic

Pharmacologic Class

opioid agonists/analgesics

Nursing Considerations

- use caution with head trauma
- can cause dizziness, headache, nausea, vomiting, respiratory depression
- do not use with MAOIs
- assess pain
- may cause respiratory in newborn
- **asses hemodynamic parameters**
- may elevate pancreatic enzymes
- **Narcan (naloxone) is the antidote**

Naproxen

Generic Name

naproxen

Trade Name

Aleve

Indication

pain, dysmenorrhea, fever, inflammation

Action

inhibits prostaglandin synthesis

Therapeutic Class

nonsteroidal anti-inflammatory agents, nonopioid analgesics, antipyretics

Pharmacologic Class

Nursing Considerations

- use caution with GI bleeding
- may increase risk for stroke and MI
- **can cause GI bleeding, anaphylaxis, Steven's Johnson syndrome**
- aspirin can decrease blood levels and effectiveness
- assess pain
- patients should remain up-right for 30 minutes after administration

Nifedipine

Generic Name

nifedipine

Trade Name

Procardia

Indication

hypertension, angina, migraines, CHF

Action

blocks calcium transport resulting in inhibition of contraction causing systemic vasodilatation

Therapeutic Class

antianginals, antihypertensives

Pharmacologic Class

Ca Channel Blocker

Nursing Considerations

- use caution in heart block, decreased blood pressure
- **don't consume grapefruit juice** while taking medication
- may cause arrhythmias
- may cause elevated liver function tests
- may cause gingival hyperplasia, Steven's Johnson syndrome
- monitor blood pressure and pulse
- monitor calcium levels
- **instruct patient on taking heart rate and blood pressure**

Nitroprusside

Generic Name

nitroprusside

Trade Name

Nitropress

Indication

hypertensive crisis, cardiogenic shock

Action

peripheral vasodilation of arteries and veins decreasing preload and afterload

Therapeutic Class

antihypertensive

Pharmacologic Class

vasodilator

Nursing Considerations

- monitor HR, BP, and EKG continuously during therapy
- may cause cyanide toxicity
- sympathomimetics may decrease effectiveness
- PAOP monitoring may help with MI and CHF patients

Norepinephrine

Generic Name

norepinephrine

Trade Name

Levophed

Indication

treatment of severe hypotension and shock

Action

increase blood pressure and cardiac output by stimulating alpha-adrenergic receptors in the blood vessels, demonstrates minor beta activity

Therapeutic Class

vasopressor

Nursing Considerations

- **monitor BP continuously if possible or every couple of minutes**
- double check all concentrations with additional nurse
- may result in rebound hypotension due to tissue ischemia when discontinued
- **monitor EKG and CVP**
- if patient is awake instruct them to report headaches, dizziness, or chest pain

Nystatin

Generic Name

nystatin

Trade Name

Mycostatin

Indication

candidiasis, denture stomatitis

Action

causes leakage of fungal cell contents

Therapeutic Class

Antifungal

Pharmacologic Class

Nursing Considerations

- may cause diarrhea, nausea, vomiting
- can be used to soak dentures
- assess mucus membrane

Olanzapine

Generic Name

olanzapine

Trade Name

Zyprexa

Indication

schizophrenia, mania, depression, anorexia nervosa, nausea/vomiting related to chemotherapy

Action

antagonizes dopamine and serotonin

Therapeutic Class

antipsychotic, mood stabilizers

Pharmacologic Class

thienobenzodiazepines

Nursing Considerations

- do not use while breastfeeding
- can cause neurolyptic malignant syndrome, seizures, suicidal thoughts, insomnia, tardive dyskinesia, agranulocytosis, constipation, tremors
- assess mental status
- monitor hemodynamics
- assess blood sugars
- assess intake and output
- monitor liver function tests

Omeprazole

Generic Name

omeprazole

Trade Name

Prilosec

Indication

GERD, ulcers, Zollinger-Ellison syndrome, reduce the risk of GI bleed in critically ill patients, heart burn

Action

prevents the transport of H ions into the gastric lumen by binding to gastric parietal cells, ↓ gastric acid production

Therapeutic Class

antiulcer agent

Pharmacologic Class

proton-pump inhibitor

Nursing Considerations

- **take 30-60 minutes prior to eating**
- capsules should be swallowed whole
- instruct patient to report black tarry stool

Ondansetron

Generic Name

ondansetron

Trade Name

Zofran

Indication

nausea/vomiting

Action

blocks effects of serotonin on vagal nerve and CNS

Therapeutic Class

antiemetic

Pharmacologic Class

5-HT3 antagonist

Nursing Considerations

- **administer slowly over 2-5 minutes - fatal QT prolongation and VTach, respiratory arrest**
- may cause headache, constipation, diarrhea, dry mouth
- asses nausea and vomiting
- **assess for extrapyramidal symptoms**
- monitor liver function tests

Oxycodone

Generic Name

oxycodone

Trade Name

Oxycontin

Indication

pain

Action

binds to opiate receptors in CNS altering the perception and sensation of pain

Therapeutic Class

Opioid Analgesic

Pharmacologic Class

opioid agonists, opioid agonists/nonopioid, analgesic combinations

Nursing Considerations

- may cause **respiratory depression**, constipation, confusion , sedation, hallucinations, urinary retention
- use caution with increased intracranial pressure
- don't use with MAOIs
- **assess hemodynamics**
- assess pain
- may elevate pancreatic enzymes
- can cause physical dependence
- assess bowel function

Oxytocin

Generic Name

oxytocin

Trade Name

Pitocin

Indication

labor induction, postpartum bleeding

Action

stimulates uterine smooth muscle

Therapeutic Class

hormones

Pharmacologic Class

oxytocics

Nursing Considerations

- can cause ICH in fetus
- can cause asphyxia in fetus
- may cause coma and seizures in mother
- may cause painful contractions
- assess fetus
- assess contractions
- monitor blood pressure
- assess maternal electrolytes
- **may cause uterine tetany**

Pancrelipase

Generic Name

pancrelipase

Trade Name

Creon

Indication

pancreatic insufficiency, ductal obstruction

Action

replacement of pancreatic enzymes: lipase, amylase, protease

Therapeutic Class

digestive agent

Pharmacologic Class

pancreatic enzyme

Nursing Considerations

- **contraindicated with pig products allergy**
- can cause shortness of breath, nausea, diarrhea, rash
- assess nutritional status
- monitor for steatorrhea
- may increase uric acid levels
- instruct patient to follow diet
- **take with meals and snacks**

Pantoprazole

Generic Name

pantoprazole

Trade Name

Protonix

Indication

GERD, heartburn, reduce the risk of GI bleed in critically ill patients

Action

prevents the transport of H ions into the gastric lumen by binding to gastric parietal cells, ↓ gastric acid production

Therapeutic Class

antiulcer agents

Pharmacologic Class

proton-pump inhibitors

Nursing Considerations

- can cause hyperglycemia, abdominal pain
- decreases absorption of certain drugs
- may increase bleeding with warfarin
- assess for occult blood
- assess liver enzymes
- assess symptoms of heart burn
- administer slowly via IV push

Paroxetine

Generic Name

paroxetine

Trade Name

Paxil

Indication

major depressive disorder, OCD, anxiety, PTSD

Action

block reuptake of serotonin in CNS

Therapeutic Class

antianxiety agent, antidepressant

Pharmacologic Class

SSRI

Nursing Considerations

- **do not use with MAOIs**
- can cause neurolyptic malignant syndrome, suicidal thoughts, serotonin syndrome, constipation, diarrhea, insomnia
- decrease effectiveness of digoxin
- increase bleeding with warfarin
- assess for suicidal thoughts

Phenazopyridine

Generic Name

phenazopyridine

Trade Name

Pyridium

Indication

urological pain

Action

provides analgesia to the urinary tract mucosa

Therapeutic Class

nonopioid analgesics

Pharmacologic Class

urinary tract analgesics

Nursing Considerations

- **will turn urine red or orange**
- may cause headache, vertigo, hepatic toxicity
- monitor renal function

Phenytoin

Generic Name

phenytoin

Trade Name

Dilantin

Indication

tonic clonic seizures, arrhythmias, neuropathic pain

Action

interferes with ion transport, shortens action potentials and decreases automaticity blocks sustained high frequency repetitive firing of action potentials.

Therapeutic Class

antiarrhythmics, anticonvulsants

Pharmacologic Class

hydantoins

Nursing Considerations

- **monitor serum phenytoin levels**
- **therapeutic levels 10-20 mcg/mL**
- use cautiously in all patients
- can cause suicidal thoughts, ataxia, extrapyramidal symptoms, hypotension, tachycardia, arrhythmias, gingival hyperplasia, nausea, rash, drug induced hepatitis, agranulocytosis, Steven's Johnson syndrome
- concurrent administration of enteral feedings may decrease absorption
- monitor for hypersensitivity
- assess seizures
- assess hemodynamics

Procainamide

Generic Name

procainamide

Indication

wide variety ventricular and atrial arrhythmias, PAC, PVC, VTach, post cardioversion

Action

decreases excitability and slows conduction velocity through the heart

Therapeutic Class

antiarrhythmic (Class IA Na Channel Blocker)

Nursing Considerations

- **may cause ventricular arrhythmias, seizure, asystole, heart block**
- monitor EKG continuously may cause widening of QRS complex
- may cause hypotension keep patient supine
- monitor for signs of agranulocytosis monitor CBC frequently
- can cause drug induced lupus syndrome

Promethazine

Generic Name

promethazine

Trade Name

Promethacon

Indication

allergic reactions, nausea and vomiting, sedation

Action

Blocks the effects of histamine, histamine plays a role in the immune response. Plays an inhibitory role on the chemoreceptor trigger zone in the medulla leading to an antiemetic effect. Possess anticholinergic properties producing CNS depression.

Therapeutic Class

antiemetic, antihistamine, sedative/hypnotic

Pharmacologic Class

phenothiazine

Nursing Considerations

- IV administration may cause damage to tissue, hypertension, impaired liver function
- monitor for neuroleptic malignant syndrome, confusion, sedation
- may cause CNS depression
- assess sedation level and anticholinergic effects

Propofol

Generic Name

propofol

Trade Name

Diprivan

Indication

anesthesia, induction, sedation,

Action

hypnotic, produces amnesia with no analgesic properties

Therapeutic Class

general anesthetic

Pharmacologic Class

Nursing Considerations

- use cautiously with CVD, lipid disorder, increased ICP
- **can cause apnea, bradycardia, hypotension**
- burning and pain at insertion site
- **can turn urine green**
- assess respiratory status and hemodynamics
- maintain patent airway
- assess level of sedation

Propranolol

Generic Name

propranolol

Trade Name

Inderal

Indication

hypertension, angina, arrythmias, cardiomyopathy, alcohol withdrawal, anxiety

Action

blocks Beta 1 and 2 adrenergic receptors

Therapeutic Class

antianginal, antiarrhythimic (class II beta blockers), antihypertensive, headache suppressant

Pharmacologic Class

beta blocker

Nursing Considerations

- contraindicated in CHF, pulmonary edema, cardiogenic shock, bradycardia, heart block
- monitor hemodynamic parameters (HR, BP)
- may cause bradycardia, CHF, pulmonary edema
- masks symptoms associated with diabetes mellitus
- advise to change positions slowly to prevent orthostatic hypotension
- instruct patient on how to take blood pressure
- stopping abruptly may result in life threatening arrhythmias
- monitor daily intake and output
- advise patient to notify physician for difficulty breathing

Propylthiouracil

Generic Name

propylthiouracil

Trade Name

PTU

Indication

hyperthyroidism

Action

inhibits thyroid hormones

Therapeutic Class

Antithyroid Agent

Pharmacologic Class

Nursing Considerations

- hepatotoxicity, nausea, vomiting, agranulocytosis
- monitor symptoms of hyperthyroidism
- monitor for hypothyroidism
- monitor WBC and liver function tests
- weight patient frequently
- may cause leukopenia, thrombocytopenia, jaundice
- take with meals

Quetiapine

Generic Name

quetiapine

Trade Name

Seroquel

Indication

schizophrenia, depressive disorder, mania

Action

dopamine and serotonin antagonist

Therapeutic Class

antipsychotic, mood stabilizers

Pharmacologic Class

Nursing Considerations

- may cause neurolyptic malignant syndrome, seizures, dizziness, palpitations, weight gain, anorexia
- **QT interval prolongation**
- don't use with CNS depressants
- assess weight frequently
- monitor liver function test and CBC
- may increase cholesterol

Ranitidine

Generic Name

ranitidine

Trade Name

Zantac

Indication

duodenal ulcers, GERD, heartburn, esophagitis, GI bleed

Action

inhibits action of histamine in gastric parietal cells, decreases gastric acid secretion

Therapeutic Class

antiulcer agents

Pharmacologic Class

histamine H2 antagonists

Nursing Considerations

- may cause arrhythmias, agranulocytosis, aplastic anemia, confusion
- assess abdominal pain
- monitor for blood in stool
- monitor CBC

Rifampin

Generic Name

rifampin

Trade Name

Rimactane

Indication

tuberculosis

Action

inhibits RNA synthesis

Therapeutic Class

Antitubercular

Pharmacologic Class

rifamycins

Nursing Considerations

- **can turn body fluids red**
- may cause diarrhea, nausea, vomiting, confusion
- assess lung sounds and sputum characteristics
- evaluate renal and liver function tests
- instruct patient not to skip or double dose
- **must complete entire dose (6-12 month therapy)**

Salmeterol

Generic Name

salmeterol

Trade Name

Serevent

Indication

reversible airway obstruction, exercise induced asthma

Action

bronchodilation through stimulation of beta 2 adrenergic receptors

Therapeutic Class

bronchodilators

Pharmacologic Class

adrenergics

Nursing Considerations

- instruct patient to avoid excessive use
- can cause headache palpitations tachycardia, abdominal pain, paradoxical bronchospasm
- beta blockers and decrease effectiveness
- assess respiratory status
- may increase glucose levels
- **always take bronchodialtor first**

Sertraline

Generic Name

sertraline

Trade Name

Zoloft

Indication

major depressive disorder, OCD, anxiety

Action

inhibits uptake of serotonin allowing for higher quantities available within synaptic cleft

Therapeutic Class

Antidepressant

Pharmacologic Class

SSRI

Nursing Considerations

- **do not use with MAOIs**
- can cause neurolyptic malignant syndrome, suicidal thoughts, drowsiness, insomnia, diarrhea, dry mouth, tremors, serotonin syndrome, sexual dysfunction
- monitor mood changes in patient
- takes 1-4 weeks for therapy to be effective.

Spironolactone

Generic Name

spironolactone

Trade Name

Aldactone

Indication

potassium loss, hypertension, edema, CHF

Action

inhibits sodium reabsorption while sparing potassium and hydrogen

Therapeutic Class

Diuretics

Pharmacologic Class

potassium sparing diuretics

Nursing Considerations

- contraindicated with hyperkalemia
- monitor intake and output
- monitor blood pressure
- **monitor potassium levels and renal panel**

Streptokinase

Generic Name

streptokinase

Trade Name

Streptase

Indication

pulmonary embolism, DVT, occluded lines, arterial thrombus

Action

converts plasminogen to plasmin which degrades fibrin clots

Therapeutic Class

Thrombolytic

Pharmacologic Class

plasminogen activators

Nursing Considerations

- contraindicated with active bleeding, hypersensitivity, bronchospasm, intracranial hemorrhage, hypotension
- begin therapy as soon as possible
- **monitor vital signs continuously**
- monitor closely for bleeding
- monitor hemodynamics
- **avoid invasive procedures**

Sucralfate

Generic Name

sucralfate

Trade Name

Carafate

Indication

management of GI ulcers, GI injury prevention from high dose aspirin and NSAID treatment

Action

reacts with gastric acid to form a paste that adheres to ulcer

Therapeutic Class

antiulcer agent

Pharmacologic Class

GI protectant

Nursing Considerations

- use caution in renal failure patients
- concurrent use of antacids may decrease the effect of sucralfate - administer 30 min before or after
- **administer on empty stomach 1 hour before meals**

Tertbutaline

Generic Name

terbutaline

Trade Name

Brethaire

Indication

asthma, COPD, preterm labor

Action

produces bronchodilation and inhibits hypersensitivity reactions

Therapeutic Class

bronchodilators

Pharmacologic Class

adrenergics

Nursing Considerations

- may cause nervousness, restlessness, tremors
- beta blockers can reduce effect
- assess respiratory status
- **monitor maternal/fetal vital signs if using for preterm labor**
- monitor for hypoglycemia
- may cause decreased potassium level

Tetracycline

Generic Name

tetracycline

Trade Name

Doxycycline

Indication

treatment of infection, gonorrhea and syphilis with penicillin allergy, chronic bronchitis

Action

bacteriostatic by inhibiting protein synthesis

Therapeutic Class

anti-infectives

Pharmacologic Class

Tetracyclines

Nursing Considerations

- use caution with liver impairment
- may cause pseudomembranous colitis, diarrhea, nausea, vomiting, photosensitivity, rash
- may increase effects of warfarin
- assess for infection
- obtain culture prior to initiating therapy
- monitor renal and liver labs
- instruct patient to complete entire dose

Trimethoprim/sulfamethoxazole

Generic Name

trimethoprim/sulfamethoxazole

Trade Name

Bactrim/TMP-SMZ

Indication

bronchitis, UTI, diarrhea, pneumonia, multiple types of infection

Action

bacteriacidal by preventing metabolism of folic acid

Therapeutic Class

anti-infectives, antiprotozoals

Pharmacologic Class

folate antagonists, sulfonamides

Nursing Considerations

- may cause renal damage, Steven Johnsons Syndrome - rash, pseudomembranous colitis, nausea, vomiting, diarrhea, rash, agranulocytosis, aplastic anemia, phlebitis
- contraindicated with sulfa allergies
- monitor CBC
- **obtain cultures prior to initiating therapy**
- monitor intake and output
- instruct patient to complete dose
- drink 8-10 glasses of water

Vancomycinn

Generic Name

vancomycin

Trade Name

Vancocin

Indication

life threatening infections, sepsis

Action

bactericidal

Therapeutic Class

anti-infectives

Pharmacologic Class

Nursing Considerations

* can cause **ototoxicity**, nausea, vomiting, nephrotoxicity, anaphylaxis, red-man syndrome
* assess for infection
* obtain culture prior to initiating therapy
* monitor blood pressure
* **dose dependent draw serum trough levels frequently**
* administer over at least 60 minutes to avoid skin irritation

Vasopressin

Generic Name

vasopressin

Trade Name

Pitressin

Indication

management of diabetes insipidus, VT/VF unresponsive to initial shock, GI hemorrhage

Action

increases water permeability of the kidney's collecting duct and distal convoluted tubule leading to water retention, also increases peripheral vascular resistance leading to increased BP

Therapeutic Class

hormone

Pharmacologic Class

antidiuretic hormone

Nursing Considerations

- use caution with HF and CV disease
- contraindicated in renal failure and hypersensitivity to pork
- monitor BP, HR, and EKG during therapy
- **monitor urine specific gravity and osmolality**
- weigh patient and assess for edema
- monitor electrolyte panel
- do not use with alcohol

Verapamil

Generic Name

verapamil

Trade Name

Isoptin

Indication

hypertension, angina, SVT, migraine

Action

prevents transport of calcium, leading to decreased contraction, decreases SA and AV node conduction

Therapeutic Class

antianginals, antiarrhythmic, antihypertensive, vascular headache suppressants

Pharmacologic Class

Ca Channel Blocker

Nursing Considerations

- **don't use with 2nd and 3rd degree heartblock**
- don't use with systolic BP < 90
- may cause anxiety, confusion, cough, dyspnea, arrhythmias, CHF, bradycardia, hypotension, elevated liver enzymes, Steven's Johnson syndrome, hyperglycemia, gingival hyperplasia
- grapefruit juice can increase effects
- can increase levels of digoxin
- monitor heart rhythm, intake and output, blood pressure
- assess angina

Warfarin

Generic Name

warfarin

Trade Name

Coumadin

Indication

venous thrombosis, pulmonary embolism, A-fib, myocardial infarction

Action

disrupts liver synthesis of Vitamin K dependent clotting factors

Therapeutic Class

Anticoagulant

Pharmacologic Class

coumarins

Nursing Considerations

* contraindicated with bleeding, severe hypertension
* can cause bleeding
* aspirin and NSAIDs can increase risk of bleeding
* azole antifungals increase effects of warfarin
* cimetadine(Tagamet) increases warfarin levels
* obtain full history of supplements and herbs
* large amounts of vitamin K may antagonize effects of warfarin
* assess for signs of bleeding
* **therapeutic levels: PT 1.3-1.5, INR 2.5-3.5**
* **instruct patient to report any signs of bleeding**
* patient should not drink alcohol
* bleeding times need to be monitored frequently

- **vitamin K is antidote**

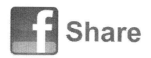

Review Now amazon

168

Common Medication Classes

ACE Inhibitors

Angiotensin-converting enzyme (ACE) inhibitors are a type of drug class most often used to lower blood pressure by relaxing blood vessels. ACE Inhibitors work by causing the body to block the production of a hormone known as angiotensin II by inhibiting the angiotensin-converting enzyme.

Angiotensin II, found naturally in the body, constricts blood vessels and releases a hormone that elevates blood pressure. The hormone also reduces the amount of water re-absorbed by the kidneys. These drugs also work in the body by decreasing the conversion of angiotensin I to angiotensin II, hence their name.

Decreasing levels of angiotensin II causes the blood vessels to dilate and for less water to be put back into the blood by the kidneys, reducing blood pressure. Some common ACE Inhibitors include: captopril, enalapril, fosinopril, imidapril, lisinopril, perindopril, ramipril, and trandolapril.

ACE Inhibitors are typically taken once a day and may be prescribed by a doctor for some of the following conditions: high blood pressure (hypertension), heart failure, kidney disease, diabetes, heart attacks, coronary artery disease, scleroderma, and migraines. Doctors may prescribe calcium channel blockers and diuretics in addition to drugs in this class. ACE inhibitors should not be taken by women that are pregnant or planning to become pregnant, as they can cause birth defects.

ACE Inhibitors are commonly prescribed by doctors because of their uncommon and mild side effects. Side effects may include: dry cough, increased blood potassium levels (hyperkalemia), fatigue, dizziness, headaches, rapid heartbeat, and fainting. In rare cases, particularly with those of African descent and tobacco users, use of ACE Inhibitors has been tied to angioedema, or swelling of the tissue. This can be life threatening if the tissues in the throat swell. Repeated use of NSAIDs (nonsteroidal anti-inflammatory drugs) such as Ibuprofen, Advil, and Motrin IB in addition to naproxen (Aleve) can decrease the effectiveness of ACE Inhibitors.

Questions about ACE Inhibitors:
1. What are some of the contraindications of the use of ACE Inhibitors?
2. How do ACE Inhibitors specifically work to lower blood pressure?
3. What are some potential side-effects that should be monitored in patients taking ACE Inhibitors?

Angiotension II Receptor Blockers

The cardiovascular system reacts in various ways to the natural Angiotensin II in the body. Angiotensin II is a potent chemical that causes contraction of muscles that surround blood vessels. Blood vessels narrow. The narrowing causes increased blood pressure. The heart is forced to work harder. Amounts of water and sodium caused by a hormone that Angiotensin II starts to release also cause increased blood pressure. Blood vessels and heart walls thicken and stiffen due to Angiotensin II.

Angiotensin II receptor blockers relax blood vessels. The heart pumps blood more effortlessly. As the blood vessels relax, blood pressure lowers. The use of Angiotensin II receptor blockers blocks the action of Angiotensin II. The blockers prevent binding to receptors on blood vessels. Blood vessels widen or dilate.

Listed here are conventional Angiotensin II receptor blockers and their trade names. The condition being treated and the health of the patient determine the best choice.

· Candesartan (Atacand)
· Irbesartan (Avapro)
· Olmesartan (Benicar)
· Losartan (Cozaar)
· Valsartan (Diovan)
· Azilsartan (Edarbi)
· Temisartan (Mecardis)
· Eprosartan (Teveten)

Indications for Use

Conditions that merit prescribing Angiotensin II receptor blockers include thickening and hardening of the skin, known as scleroderma. They are beneficial when prescribed for chronic kidney diseases, diabetic renal failure, heart failure and high blood pressure. Kidney disease progression due to diabetes or high blood pressure diminishes. Reduced risk of stroke or diabetes prevention is possible in high blood pressure patients. Patients who cannot tolerate ACE (angiotensin-converting-enzyme) inhibitors are often prescribed Angiotensin II receptor blockers because they produce similar effects.

Side Effects

Very few people suffer from Angiotensin II receptor blocker side effects. Those who do, report bouts of

· Diarrhea
· Leg and back pain
· Nasal congestion
· Lightheadedness
· Dizziness
· Headaches.

Some people taking Olmesartan reported sprue-like enteropathy that is an intestinal problem. Other rare, but serious, side effects are angioedema (localized tissue swelling), white blood cell drop, allergic reaction, liver failure, and kidney failure. Women planning a pregnancy, or are already pregnant should not take Angiotensin II receptor blockers. They are a possible cause of birth defects.

Questions:

When are Angiotensin II receptor blockers prescribed?
How do Angiotensin II receptor blockers work?
What are possible side effects of Angiotensin II receptor blockers?

Antianginals

Antianginals are used to manage the pain of angina. They act by either reducing the oxygen needs of the heart or by improving the oxygen flow to the heart, or both. There are three major classes of antianginals and three different types of angina.

Stable angina is caused by a partial occlusion of a coronary artery. Unstable angina is due to the rupture of an atherosclerotic plaque. Variant angina is due to vasospasm of coronary arteries.

Beta-adrenoreceptor antagonists

These drugs reduce the heart rate, which reduces the metabolic needs of the heart. They are used to prevent attacks of stable angina due to exertion. They block the beta receptors and keep the heart rate down below the point at which pain occurs.

Beta blockers are indicated as a first-line treatment for stable angina. They are often used in combination with calcium blockers. Beta blockers are contradicted in variant angina and in people with severe asthma. They should be used cautiously in diabetics because they can cause hypoglycemia.

Organic nitrates

These drugs are vasodilators that improve perfusion of the heart. They stimulate the endothelium-derived relaxing factor that dilates the veins and reduces pressure in the ventricles. Both of these mechanisms of action reduce oxygen requirements of the heart muscle.

Nitrates are taken both for immediate relief of painful stable angina attacks and as maintenance therapy to prevent future attacks. However, long-term maintenance nitrate use may cause increased oxidative stress and endothelial dysfunction and may not be safe.

Calcium antagonists

Calcium blockers, or antagonists, dilate blood vessels, improve heart efficiency and reduce the heart rate. Calcium blockers come in three different classes. Class I blockers have a strong negative inotropic effect. Class II blockers do not affect the conductivity or contractions of the heart. Class III blockers have no inotropic effects.

Calcium blockers are used to treat stable angina and variant angina. For treating stable angina, they can be used alone or in combination with beta blockers.

Study Questions

1. Which class of drug is used to abort angina attacks?
2. Which class of drug can cause hypoglycemia in diabetics?
3. Which two classes of drugs are often used together to treat stable angina?

Antidysrhythmics

Antidysrythmic drugs are commonly used to treat dysrhythmias. A dysrhythmia is an abnormal heart beat, and these drugs can help to correct any abnormalities. There are four different classes of drugs that medical professionals should consider when administering the drugs. Here are some details of the four classes and the contraindications.

Classes of Antidysrhythmic

Class I:

Class I drugs are known for interacting with the **sodium channels**. This class is further subdivided into a, b, or c class.

Class II:

Class II drugs are **beta-blockers** and work by reducing the sympathetic nervous system stimulation associated with the heart. Impulses in the heart are also reduced or blocked with impulse and transmissions. They work by blocking the effects of catecholamines. If you need to treat supraventricular tachycardias, these drugs are particularly useful.

Class III:

Class III drugs increase the APD through the prolonging of repolarization. These drugs will block **potassium channels**, but will not affect the conduction velocity. The combination of these two actions will prevent any re-entrant arrhythmias. "Class III agents have the potential to prolong the QT interval of the EKG."

Class IV:

Class IV drugs inhibit the **calcium channels** by reducing the movement of calcium ions during action potentials. Cardiac action potential is shortened when the conduction through the AV node is decreased. Adrenergic control of heart rate and contractility is controlled through Class IV drugs, which include verapamil or diltiazem.

Adverse Effects

Some common reactions include nausea, diarrhea, vomiting, blurred vision, and headache. Even some antiarrhythmics are known for causing dysrhythmias. Drug toxicity is another adverse effect. Antidysrhythmic drugs involve circulation, CNS, and the heart.

Contraindications

All known drug allergies should be included in addition to cardiogenic shock, major ECG changes, sick sinus syndrome, and bundle branch block.

Interactions

Anticoagulant activity with warfarin is a strong potential with these types of drugs.

Antidysrythmics are important to any medical professional treating patients with irregular heartbeats and other abnormalities associated with heart rhythms. When used properly the drugs are effective. Consider the use of antidysrhythmics to alleviate symptoms in patients who are experiencing related health conditions.

Antiemetics
Medications that help to control nausea and vomiting from a variety of illnesses and conditions are called antiemetics. These medications help to calm the sensations that lead to repeated vomiting and that can lead to fluid loss and severe dehydration. However, these drugs do not treat the underlying medical condition that is causing the nausea and vomiting. A number of different drug classes are used to control nausea and vomiting, including dopamine antagonists, anticholinergics, antihistamines and others.

How Antiemetic Medications Work
Nausea and vomiting are caused by stimulation of the vomiting center in the medulla of the brain. Each class of antiemetic drug works in a different way:

· **Anticholinergics** – These drugs reduce the action of acetylcholine at the muscarinic receptor of the brain. Dimenhydrinate, diphenhydramine, scopolamine and meclizine are examples of these medications.

· **Antihistamines** – These drugs inhibit the action of histamine at the H1 receptor in the brain. Metroclopromide, promethazine and doxylamine are examples of these drugs.

· **Dopamine antagonists** – These drugs work by minimizing the effect of dopamine at the D2 receptor in the chemoreceptor trigger zone of the medulla. Prochlorperazine, chlorpromazine and phenothiazine are examples of this type of medication.

Indications For Use
Antiemetic medications are used for a number of conditions. They are frequently used for severe nausea and vomiting that occurs with pregnancy. Antiemetics are also useful in controlling symptoms of gastrointestinal problems caused by viruses, food poisoning or other issues. Antiemetics are important medications for relieving the nausea and vomiting related to chemotherapy and other cancer treatments. Nausea and vomiting can also occur after surgery, as a result of the effects of anesthesia.

Side Effects
Most side effects from antiemetic medications are minor and are outweighed by the value of the medication for patients. Generally, these side effects fade after a period of use. Side effects include:

· Dry mouth

· Sensitivity to sunlight

· Stuffy nose

· Constipation

However, if more severe side effects, the patient should receive further medical attention immediately:

· Hives

· Fever

· Swelling of lips

· Vision problems

· Uncontrollable facial or body movements

· Fainting

· Trembling

· Sweating

· Problems with breathing

· Seizures

· Loss of bladder control

Antidepressants

Antidepressants are used to treat a number of symptoms and conditions. These drugs work to create balanced chemical levels in the brain's neurotransmitters, in order to reduce symptoms of depression or anxiety disorders.

Neurotransmitters link cells, providing communication within the brain. Neurotransmitters are released by a certain nerve and taken up by others; however, when they are not collected by another nerve, they are taken back by the original nerve - a process called "reuptake". The neurotransmitters commonly linked to depression are serotonin, dopamine and norepinephrine.

TYPES OF ANTIDEPRESSANTS
There are a few main types of antidepressants. These include:

Tricyclic (or tetracyclic) antidepressants (TCAs) - Called cyclic antidepressants in general, and categorized by the number of rings in their chemical makeup; three (tri) or four (tetra). These were among the first antidepressants created, but have been widely replaced by more common types (with less side effects). However, they have been found to be successful in certain cases where other antidepressants were not.

Selective serotonin reuptake inhibitors (SSRIs) - Because these particular antidepressants cause fewer side effects than the others, they are the kind that are most often prescribed.

Monoamine oxidase inhibitors (MAOIs) - The first antidepressants created, but they are being used less often because of the possible side effects and dietary restrictions. Because of the risk of high blood pressure, certain foods that may interact with this medication must be limited.

Side Effects

Though they are different types, these antidepressants are used to treat the same disorders and symptoms, and generally have similar side effects. These effects may include: Dry mouth; dizziness; blurred vision; drowsiness; constipation; headache; anxiety; insomnia; nausea or vomiting; sexual dysfunction; seizures; and more. While each type of antidepressant has its own specific side effects, the number is quite small compared to the number that all three types have in common.

Indications for Use

178

The FDA outlines indications for use (conditions for which they are prescribed to treat) for drugs. Antidepressant indications for use typically include: Anxiety disorders; obsessive-compulsive disorder (OCD); panic disorder (PD); post-traumatic stress disorder (PTSD); anorexia and bulimia; personality disorders; attention deficit hyperactivity disorder (ADHD); and several other disorders and/or conditions.

QUESTIONS
What are the three main types of antidepressants used?
What are the neurotransmitters in the brain that are linked to depression?

Antiplatelet Medications

General Information: Antiplatelet drugs are a class of medications that inhibit thrombus (blood clot) formation.

Indications: Antiplatelet drugs are primarily used to treat and/or prevent thromboembolic ischemic events such as stroke or myocardial infarction. They are commonly prescribed to patients who have had cardiac stents placed. Antiplatelet drugs can be paired with thrombolytic (tPA) and/or anticoagulant medications (heparin, warfarin) either to treat acute events or for long-term prevention.

Commonly used antiplatelet drugs include aspirin (ASA), clopidogrel (Plavix), prasugrel (Effient), dipyridamole (Persantine, Aggrenox), and ticagrelor (Brilinta).

Mechanism of Action: Antiplatelet drugs all work by decreasing the platelets' ability to stick to one another and form a clot, called aggregation. Aspirin indirectly inhibits the production of thromboxane, a substance important for clot formation. Clopidogrel, ticagrelor, and prasugrel all bind to and block a receptor called P2Y12, which is involved in the activation of platelets and cross-linkage with fibrin. It is important to know that some antiplatelet drugs, including aspirin, clopidogrel, and prasugrel, bind irreversibly to the platelet; their effects persist for the 7-10 day lifespan of the cell. Newer drugs like ticagrelor have the advantage of binding reversibly, and their effects will wear off within hours of discontinuation of the medication.

Side Effects and Precautions: Because they decrease the body's ability to form blood clots, antiplatelet drugs make bleeding a serious risk for patients taking them. This is especially true for those who concurrently take NSAIDs, thrombolytics, or anticoagulants. Other side effects vary from drug to drug. Caution should be used in patients with a history of GI bleeds or ulcers, or at other risk for bleeding (recent trauma or surgery). Safety has not been established in pregnant or lactating mothers or children. If patients require surgery, discontinuation of antiplatelet drugs is often recommended 7-10 days prior.

Monitoring: Periodic lab monitoring of bleeding time should be performed during therapy.

Patient Education: Teach patients signs of bleeding including CNS/hemorrhagic stroke symptoms. Ensure that patients understand the need for immediate medical attention if signs or symptoms of bleeding are observed.

Questions:

1. Why would a patient with newly placed coronary stents be prescribed an antiplatelet drug?
2. What are some signs and symptoms of bleeding that patients on antiplatelet drugs should be aware of?
3. Why is it recommended that patients discontinue taking aspirin one week before having surgery?

Benzodiazepines

Benzodiazepines are used as sedatives, hypnotics, anxiolytics, muscle relaxants and anticonvulsants. They act by enhancing the response of gamma-aminobutyric acid-A (GABA-A) receptors to GABA, a neurotransmitter. Neurons affected by benzodiazepines become resistant to excitation. Benzodiazepines come in short-term, moderate-term and long-acting forms. They can be taken orally or in injectable or rectal forms.

Indications
Indications for treatment with benzodiazepines include sedation, seizures, insomnia, anxiety, agitation, alcohol withdrawal, and muscle spasms. It is unclear if benzodiazepines are safe during pregnancy. Alcohol should be avoided when using benzodiazepines.

In health-care settings, benzodiazepines are commonly used for their sedating properties. They are used in intensive care settings with patients experiencing extreme distress. They are commonly given before medical or dental procedures to relieve anxiety- in this use, they can also cause amnesia, so the patient doesn't recall any unpleasant details of the procedure.

In cases of prolonged seizures, administration of fast-acting benzodiazepines is the treatment of choice.

For occasional insomnia, benzodiazepines are quite effective in inducing sleep and keeping patients asleep. They can also be used for the treatment of acute anxiety or agitation and are commonly used to ease the symptoms of alcohol withdrawal.

Side Effects
The most common side effects of benzodiazepines are drowsiness, dizziness, and decreased alertness. Driving accidents and falls are both possible problems. Less-frequent side effects include nausea, confusion and nightmares.

Safety
Benzodiazepines are considered safe for short-term use, but occasionally some individuals will experience cognitive impairment.

Some individuals respond paradoxically to benzodiazepines with agitation and panic. Elderly individuals are more likely to suffer severe side effects, including dementia, in response to benzodiazepines. Long-term use of benzodiazepines is controversial because of the development of physical and mental dependence and withdrawal symptoms if the medication is stopped abruptly. Long-term use can also cause cognitive impairment, depression and anxiety. Many guidelines suggest using benzodiazepines continuously for no longer than two to four weeks. They can be used intermittently for longer periods of time.

Abuse
Benzodiazepines are frequently abused, often in association with other drugs of abuse.

An overdose of benzodiazepine can cause deep unconsciousness but is rarely fatal on its own. However, when benzodiazepines are taken along with alcohol or opiates, the risk of a fatal reaction increases exponentially.

Study Questions
1. Which neurotransmitter receptor do benzodiazepines act upon?
2. Why is long-term use of benzodiazepines considered unsafe?
3. What are the most common side effects of benzodiazepines?

Calcium Channel Blockers

Calcium channel blockers, or calcium antagonists, relax and widen blood vessels by acting on the muscle cells in the arterial walls. They do this by preventing calcium from entering the cells of the heart and blood vessels, which in turn lowers blood pressure.

Some calcium channel blockers provide the added benefit of also slowing down heart rate, which aside from reducing blood pressure, can also relieve angina (chest pain) and help stabilize an irregular heartbeat.

Calcium channel blockers are available in both short-acting and long-acting forms. The short-acting forms distribute quickly, but their effects only last a few hours. The long-acting forms release the medication more slowly, resulting in a longer lasting effect.

Examples of calcium channel blockers include:

- Isradipine
- Amlodipine (Norvasc)
- Diltiazem (Cardizem, Tiazac)
- Felodipine
- Nicardipine (Cardene SR)
- Verapimil (Calan, Veralan, Covera-HS)
- Nifedipine (Procardia)
- Nisoldipine (Sular)

Calcium channel blockers are prescribed to help treat, prevent, or improve the symptoms of a wide variety of conditions, including:

- Arrhythmia (irregular heartbeat)
- Angina (chest pain)
- Migraine
- Brain aneurysm complications
- A number of circulatory conditions, such as Raynaud's disease
- Hypertension (High blood pressure)
- Pulmonary hypertension (High blood pressure that affects the arteries in the lungs)

Calcium channel blockers might not be as effective in lowering blood pressure as beta blockers, diuretics, or angiotensin-converting enzyme (ACE) inhibitors. Therefore, they are usually not considered a first course of treatment when treating high blood pressure. Calcium channel blockers are oftentimes prescribed along with other blood pressure medications or with statins (cholesterol-lowering drugs).

However, in the case of African-Americans, calcium channel blockers have been shown to be more effective than other blood pressure medications such as ACE inhibitors, angiotensin II receptor blockers, or beta blockers.

Some side effects of calcium channel blockers include:

- Rash
- Flushing
- Fatigue
- Nausea
- Tachycardia (rapid heartbeat)
- Headache
- Dizziness
- Constipation
- Swelling in the lower legs and feet

Certain calcium channel blockers interact negatively with grapefruit juice, the most outstanding interaction occurring while taking Felodipine. Also, some calcium channel blockers can reduce the body's ability to eliminate calcium channel blockers. The medication then builds up in the system which causes serious side effects.

Questions:

What are calcium channel blockers and how do they work?
What are some examples of calcium channel blockers?
How do calcium channel blockers affect the African-American population differently?

Cardiac Glycosides

Cardiac glycosides are a medication made of an organic molecule with a glycoside sugar. The most common one used in medicine is digoxin, also known as digitalis.

Mechanism of Cardiac Glycosides

Under normal conditions in the absence of cardiac glycoside, sodium-potassium pumps import potassium and export sodium. Another pump, the NCX exchanger, imports sodium into the cell and exports calcium. Cardiac glycosides halt the action of the sodium-potassium pump, making sodium build up in the cell. This stops the NCX pump from working because the cell is already hypernatremic. Calcium will then build up and the excess stored in the sarcoplasmic reticulum.

When released on stimulation, this excess calcium will cause a more powerful and rapid contraction. Cardiac glycosides also increase the repolarization phase of myocytes and thus increase the AV node's refractory period. In higher doses, cardiac glycosides may depress the SA node as well, which can be dangerous.

The result is more effective contraction of the heart muscle and a better regulated heart rate. Cardiac glycosides are anti-arrhythmic and increase cardiac output while reducing the heart rate.

Indications for the Use of Cardiac Glycosides

Cardiac glycosides are used mainly for congestive heart failure and atrial fibrillation. They are contraindicated in patients with ventricular fibrillation.

Side Effects

The most serious side effects of cardiac glycosides are arrhythmia, nausea and vomiting, anorexia, and blurry vision. These symptoms may also suggest toxicity. In addition, common side effects include:

- bradycardia
- loss of consciousness
- dizziness
- bleeding problems from liver toxicity
- rash
- petechiae
- abdominal pain

Because cardiac glycosides are used to treat arrhythmias but also can cause or worsen these, it is important for patients to be monitored when treatment is initiated. However, patients should seek medical care immediately if any of these side effects occur, as all can be dangerous to patients with cardiac failure and also may suggest toxicity.
Questions:

What electrolyte imbalance can mimic the effects of cardiac glycosides?

A patient is started on digoxin. A few days later, he calls his nurse to report side effects of edema, anorexia, and constipation. Which of these may suggest cardiac glycoside toxicity?

Diuretics

Diuretics, or water pills, are a classification of drugs used to treat many different conditions. They work by helping to rid the body of sodium and water by making the kidneys excrete more sodium into the urine. The sodium draws water with it from the blood which reduces the amount of fluid flowing through the blood vessels, thus reducing pressure on the artery walls.

The three main types of diuretics are **thiazide, potassium-sparing and loop**. Each works differently by affecting a different part of the kidneys.

Thiazides not only act on the kidneys, but they also help to dilate the blood vessels.

Loop diuretics make the kidneys excrete more fluid by interfering with the transport of salt and water across certain kidney cells in a structure known as the Loop of Henle, where the name is taken from.

Potassium-sparing diuretics are weak diuretics most often prescribed in combination with thiazide and loop diuretics to help prevent hypokalemia (low blood potassium).

Common thiazide diuretics include:

- Indapamide
- Chlorothiazide (Diuril)
- Hydrochlorothiazide (Microzide)
- Metolazone (Zaroxolyn)
- Chlorthalidone

Common potassium-sparing diuretics include:

- Spironolactone (Aldactone)
- Triamterene (Dyrenium)
- Amiloride
- Eplerenone (Inspra)

Common loop diuretics include:

- Furosemide (Lasix)
- Bumetanide
- Torsemide (Demadex)
- Ethacrynic Acid (Edecrin)

The type, and combination of diuretics prescribed depends on the patient's overall health and the condition being treated. Aside from high blood pressure, edema, and glaucoma, diuretics are used to treat, prevent, or improve symptoms in a range of other conditions such as:

- Heart Failure
- Kidney stones
- Polycystic ovarian disease
- Osteoporosis
- Diabetes insipidus
- Hirsutism (Male-pattern hair growth in women)

Diuretics are usually well tolerated but they do have some side effects, the most common being frequent urination with the use of loop diuretics.

Other possible side effects include:

- Hypokalemia (low blood potassium)
- Hyperkalemia (with potassium-sparing use)
- Hyponatremia (low sodium in the blood)
- Headaches
- Dizziness
- Muscle cramps
- Increased blood sugar or cholesterol
- Increased thirst
- Joint conditions such as gout
- Impotence
- Rashes
- Gynecomastia (enlargement of the breasts in men)

Questions:

What are the three main types of diuretics and how does each one work?
What conditions do diuretics treat?
What possible side effects are associated with the use of diuretics?

Insulin

Insulin is one of most important hormones in the human body. It helps to regulate the metabolism of carbohydrates and fats that are consumed. When insulin is not utilized in the body or is not produced in sufficient quantities, diabetes mellitus can result, a serious metabolic disease that can affect the function of many organs.

What Is Insulin?
Insulin is a protein produced by the human body. The word "insulin" comes from the Latin word meaning "island." Insulin is produced in the pancreas in the islets of Langherans, small areas of the pancreas that contain beta cells that produce the compound.

Insulin is produced when carbohydrate foods are ingested and convert to glucose. The insulin helps the body to store and absorb the glucose as it is needed. The insulin in different species of animal is similar to human insulin, but varies in strength. Insulin from pigs is considered to be closest in composition to human insulin.

How Does Insulin Work in the Body?
After eating, glucose in the bloodstream triggers the pancreas to release insulin. The insulin travels to the cells of the body, sending a message to open up to allow the glucose in, so that it can be used for energy or stored for later use. When the body cannot produce its own insulin, or cannot produce enough insulin, it must be introduced artificially into the body to produce this effect.

How Is Insulin Used?
Insulin comes as a solution or in suspension with particles that settle on standing. It must be injected into the body subcutaneously, that is, under the skin. Insulin may come in vials used with syringes; pre-filled disposable devices or cartridges used with insulin pens.

Indications For Use
Insulin is used to regulate blood glucose levels in patients who are not able to produce insulin, such as in Type-1 diabetes, or in patients with Type-2 diabetes whose blood glucose levels cannot be managed with other types of medication.

Side Effects of Insulin
The use of insulin sometimes causes side effects. If side effects are severe, they should be brought to the attention of the physician:

· Redness, swelling or itching at the injection site or on the body

· Skin thickening or depressions in the skin

· Weight gain

· Constipation

Severe side effects that need immediate medical attention include:

· Shortness of breath
· Wheezing
· Dizziness
· Fast heartbeat
· Sweating
· Blurred vision
· Difficulty breathing or swallowing
· Swelling of the extremities
· Muscle cramps
· Weakness

NSAIDs

Mechanism of Action

Nonsteroidal anti-inflammatory agents (NSAIDs) all act to block the cyclo-oxygenase (COX) enzymes. There are two COX enzymes. Both COX enzymes are involved in producing prostaglandins and thromboxanes. COX-1 is present in most tissues, but COX-2 is only produced in inflammatory cells and plays an essential role in inflammation.

Most NSAIDs inhibit both COX enzymes. Their desirable properties are caused by inhibition of COX-2 and most of their side effects are caused by inhibition of COX-1. Inhibition of COX-1 reduces the production of prostaglandins that protect the stomach from acid and support platelet function. As a consequence, all NSAIDs have the potential to cause stomach ulcers and reduce clotting time.

Indications

NSAIDs are used to treat mild to moderate pain and inflammation, and to reduce fevers. Headaches, arthritis pain, and pain associated with minor viral infections are the most common indications for NSAIDs. Low doses of aspirin are also used to reduce the risk of strokes and heart attack by inhibiting clotting of the blood.

Side Effects

The most common side effects of NSAIDs are gastrointestinal in nature and include nausea, reduced appetite, vomiting, diarrhea, and constipation. Some people develop headaches or dizziness. Occasionally swelling of the ankles will occur. More severe side effects include stomach ulcers, kidney failure, liver failure and prolonged bleeding. NSAIDs can also increase the risk of stroke and heart attacks, particularly in individuals already at risk for such conditions. Severe side effects are usually associated with chronic use of NSAIDs.

Warnings and Drug Interactions

Some individuals are allergic to NSAIDs. Anyone with an allergy to one NSAID is likely to be allergic to all NSAIDs.

Aspirin should not be given to children or teenagers with chickenpox or influenza due to the risk of developing Reye's syndrome.

NSAIDs may reduce the effectiveness of diuretics. Because NSAIDs inhibit clotting, they should only be used with care in individuals on anticoagulants such as warfarin.

Administration

NSAIDs are almost always given orally. The dose and frequency of dosing vary by each type of NSAID. Taking the medication with food may reduce the risk of nausea.

Study Questions

1. Which COX enzyme is responsible for protecting the stomach lining?
2. Which NSAIDs can cause stomach ulcers and prolonged bleeding?

3. Who should not be given aspirin?

An opioid is within a class of drugs that affect the opioid receptors of the brain causing a general CNS depression. In doing such, the drugs alter perception of pain. Many opioids exist, and they all resemble morphine in some fashion. The drugs are in a pregnancy risk class C, which means they cannot be ruled out as harmful substances to pregnant women.

What Are Opioids Used For?

Opioid can be used for severe pain that drugs such as acetaminophen and ibuprofen cannot alleviate alone. Opioid pills are often mixed acetaminophen or ibuprofen. The mixture of the analgesic and the narcotic gives the patient maximum pain protection.

What Are the Side Effects of Opioids?

The most common side effects of an opioids are general CNS depression which can include decrease blood pressure, pulse, and in some patients decreased respiratory drive. Patients should be monitored closely during opiate use.

Nausea is another common side effect that occurs in people who take opioid pills. Some additional side effects include vomiting, itching, sweating, hot flashes and headaches. Such effects do not occur in all patients.

194

Statins

Statins reduce cholesterol levels in the body.

This drug group targets the liver's cholesterol production by inhibiting the enzyme HMG-CoA reductase. This process replaces the HMG-CoA reductase in the liver. The decreased production of cholesterol initiates two significant occurrences. Supplementary enzymes form and create a protein that significantly increases the production of LDL. These additional receptors bind with the existing LDL and VLDL in the liver. The liver digests this fatty substance; reducing cholesterol levels.

Uses

-Atheroma and related diseases, such as heart disease and atherosclerosis
-Diabetes
-A family history of heart attacks, especially at a young age
-Increased age
-High cholesterol

Common Statins

-Atorvastatin [most potent]
-Rosuvastatin [most potent]
-Cerivastatin
-Pravastatin
-Lovastatin
-Mevastatin
-Pitavastatin
-Simvastatin
-Fluvastatin {least potent}

A single statin drug regimen can successfully reduce cholesterol levels. Sometimes a combination of a statin and niacin [niaspan or niacor] is required, as with these conditions.

High LDL and High Triglycerides
A statin drug and Fibric Acid such as, Fenofibrate {TriCor, Fenoglide} may be useful. There is an increased risk of developing muscle problems.

High Triglycerides only
*Niacin
*Fibric Acid
*Fish Oil, Omega3 fatty acids {Lovaza 2-4 gram doses}
Low HDL
*Niacin {especially if LDL remains high}
*Exercise and weight loss

Side Effects

-Muscle Aches
-Pain
-Weakness
-Neuropathy
-Hepatic and Pancreatic dysfunction
-Asymptomatic Liver damage
-Cognitive impairment [some users report memory loss, forgetfulness, and confusion]
-Elevated blood sugar levels.
-Lovastatin may interact with other patient medications.

These may indicate the development of severe complications. The physician might request the patient stop taking the medication. If the patient's condition remains unchanged, the doctor can do a more comprehensive evaluation. The physician may order blood tests, a percutaneous muscle biopsy, or genetic tests.

Questions

Can you describe the sequential process of how statins reduce cholesterol levels?
Can you list the types of statin drugs and indicate which ones are the most potent and which are the least potent?

Respiratory Drugs

Drugs that affect the respiratory system can be divided into four general categories.

Antihistamines

Antihistamines, also called H1 blockers, block histamine from binding to receptors. Histamines are released in response to allergens, irritants and general inflammation. When they bind to their receptors, they cause the airways to constrict and release secretions.

Indications for antihistamines include simple allergic reactions, such as allergic sinusitis and urticaria. They can also be helpful for treating rhinitis. Antihistamines are contradicted in pregnancy. They should only be used with caution in individuals with liver or kidney impairment, or with prolonged QT intervals.

Antihistamines come in two classes, first generation and second generation. First-generation drugs have many more side effects due to their stronger anticholinergic effects. The chief side effect to be aware of is sedation.

Decongestants

Decongestants stimulate the alpha-adrenergic receptors, which causes the blood vessels in the mucus membranes to constrict. This reduces the swelling of tissues and the production of secretions. Decongestants come in nasal spray and oral forms.

Decongestants are indicated for rhinitis, sinusitis, allergic reactions, and upper respiratory tract infections. They should only be used cautiously in patients with high blood pressure.

Side effects of decongestants include elevated blood pressure, nervousness and insomnia. Nasal sprays have fewer side effects than oral formulations, but if nasal sprays are used for more than a few days they can cause increased congestion.

Expectorants and Mucolytics

Expectorants act to help individuals clear their respiratory pathways of secretions by increasing the amount of fluid included in the secretions, causing the mucus to become less viscous. The mucolytics also help loosen and break down mucus so it is easier to cough up. They act by directly cleaving chemical bonds in the mucus to make it less viscous.

Indications for mucolytics and expectorants include upper respiratory infections, rhinitis, cystic fibrosis, chronic productive cough and pneumonia.

Side effects of mucolytics are nausea and irritation of the respiratory tract. Side effects of expectorants are nausea and vomiting.

Antitussives

Antitussives act to block the cough reflex. Most antitussives are narcotics that act directly on the nervous system to block coughing without affecting respiration.

Antitussives are indicated in cases of troublesome chronic dry cough. However, caution should be used when administering these drugs because many individuals need to cough to keep their respiratory pathways clear of secretions.

Side effects include drowsiness, nausea, and drying of the mucus membranes.

Questions
What is the primary side effect of first-generation antihistamines?
Can decongestants be given to patients with high blood pressure?
What is the difference between expectorants and mucolytics?

Beta Blockers

Beta blockers, known medically as Beta-adrenergic blocking agents, are typically prescribed for people who have suffered a heart attack or who have high blood pressure. Some common names for these medications include atenolol, acebutolol, bisoprolol, metaprolol, nadalol, and propranolol. This type of medication is usually prescribed after diuretics and other blood pressure medications do not work. They can also be combined with other types of medications called angiotensin-converting enzyme (ACE) inhibitors. According to the American Heart Association, beta blockers can help people live longer after a suffering a heart attack.

What do beta blockers do?

According to the Mayo Clinic, beta blockers block adrenaline or epinephrine. This keeps the heart beating at a slower rate than what a person is used to, and it also keeps the heart from beating as hard as it had been. Beta blockers also open up blood vessels. The combination of opening the vessels and slowing down heart rate keeps blood pressure down.

Beta blockers help reduce systolic blood pressure numbers. These types of medications are prescribed for people who have had a heart attack. They are useful for stopping or lessening angina or chest pain. Beta blockers are also used to control migraines, glaucoma, hyperthyroidism, generalized anxiety disorder, heart failure, and some types of tremors.

What are the side effects of taking beta blockers?

Some of the side effects that people can experience while on this type of medication are fatigue, upset stomach, diarrhea, constipation, and dizziness. Rarer side effects include trouble breathing, depression, loss of sex drive, and trouble sleeping. People who have asthma are not usually prescribed this type of medication due to constriction of the bronchial tubes.

Because beta blockers reduce the heart's required oxygen input. Diabetics should always monitor blood sugar carefully when prescribed beta blockers because the medication can mask the symptoms of low blood pressure like a fast heartbeat.

Speaking to the prescribing physician about exercise and how beta blockers affect the body is always recommended. People who take beta blockers should not stop taking the medication without the advice of a doctor because sudden stopping can cause a heart attack or other heart problems to occur. Taking a beta blocker may help some people tolerate exercise better than they did before they began taking the medicine.

View Other Books from NRSNG.com | NursingStudentBooks.com

200

As a Gift:
http://www.nrsng.com/50meds

Wonder which are the most commonly prescribed medications?

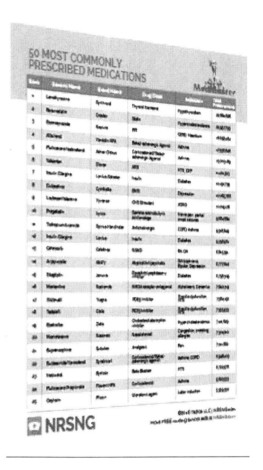

Download our free PDF cheat sheet covering the **50 Most Commonly Prescribed Medications . . . Just visit NRSNG.com/50meds**

50 Most Commonly Prescribed Med Free Cheatsheet: **NRSNG.com/50meds**
Nursing School Shouldn't be so DAMN Hard!
©2016 TazKai LLC | NRSNG.com

Search for Jon Haws and NRSNG on Amazon to find other books and resources from
NRSNG.com